GOING VEGAN

YOUR DAILY PLANNER

Everything You Need to Transition to a Vegan Diet

MICHELLE NEFF

Adams Media

New York London Toronto Sydney New Delhi

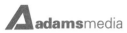

Adams Media
An Imprint of Simon & Schuster, Inc.
57 Littlefield Street
Avon, Massachusetts 02322

First Adams Media trade paperback edition December 2019

ADAMS MEDIA and colophon are trademarks of Simon & Schuster.

For information about special discounts for bulk purchases, please contact Simon & Schuster Special Sales at 1-866-506-1949 or business@simonandschuster.com.

The Simon & Schuster Speakers Bureau can bring authors to your live event. For more information or to book an event contact the Simon & Schuster Speakers Bureau at 1-866-248-3049 or visit our website at www.simonspeakers.com.

Interior design by Colleen Cunningham
Interior images by Priscilla Yuen

Manufactured in the United States of America

10 9 8 7 6 5 4 3 2 1

Library of Congress Cataloging-in-Publication Data has been applied for.

ISBN 978-1-5072-1206-6
ISBN 978-1-5072-1207-3 (ebook)

Contains material adapted from the following title published by Adams Media, an Imprint of Simon & Schuster, Inc.: *The Daily Vegan Planner: 12 Weeks to a Complete Vegan Diet Transition* by Jolinda Hackett, copyright © 2012, ISBN 978-1-4405-2998-6.

CONTENTS

INTRODUCTION

So, you're thinking of going vegan…but have no idea where to start. How do you make your favorite dishes vegan? How do you know if you're following a healthy diet and getting all the nutrients your body needs? And how do you make going vegan a long-term lifestyle change?

As you may have guessed, going vegan does require a few changes to your daily life—but not to worry! *Going Vegan: Your Daily Planner* is here to help make your transition as smooth as possible. Within this planner, you'll find everything you need to know to make your transition to a vegan diet successful for a lifetime, including information about nutrition, food labeling, vegan cooking, and even changing your shopping habits at the grocery store.

The goal of this planner is to help you become a healthy and happy vegan—and not just for the twelve weeks outlined here, but for as long as you want. By the time you're done following this twelve-week vegan meal plan, being vegan will be so easy that you'll barely even have to think about it! You'll learn how to cook simple, healthy vegan recipes that will keep you nourished, excited, and committed to a vegan diet. And thanks to well-balanced meals, you'll know with complete confidence that you're getting more than enough protein (and all the rest of your nutrients, too!) to keep your body feeling its best.

As you follow along with the planner, you'll also learn something exciting: Going vegan is fun! Each week, you'll try new foods and maybe even venture out to a different grocery store for the ingredients you'll need. You'll be supporting your body with a happy, healthy lifestyle. Your vegan lifestyle can have serious positive changes to protect the environment and animal welfare, so you can feel good about making a difference in your community too. Who knows, you might even make some new vegan friends shopping the vegan section of your local health food store!

By the end of these twelve weeks, you'll be familiar with a wide variety of vegan foods and cooking techniques, and you'll be able to prepare healthy, tasty, and well-balanced meals with confidence. Your journey to veganism starts now!

ON BECOMING VEGAN

GETTING STARTED

YOU'VE DECIDED TO GO VEGAN. NOW WHAT?

Anthropologist Margaret Mead once said, "It is easier to change a man's religion than it is to change his diet." We may eat for sustenance, for pleasure, out of boredom or mindlessness, or perhaps due to cultural reasons. At thirty years old, the average adult has eaten more than 30,000 meals in their lifetime.

Although you're cutting all animal products (and possibly foods that may have used animals in their production) from your diet, you really won't miss a thing. As a vegan, a nearly infinite myriad of grains, herbs, fruits, vegetables, beans, and legumes from around the world is at your fingertips. Plus, you'll find countless animal and dairy alternative products at your local grocery store. For instance, there is a plethora of dairy-free cheeses available from companies such as Daiya, Miyoko's, and Follow Your Heart. Similarly, there is no shortage of meat-free alternatives from companies like Beyond Meat, Gardein, Lightlife, Tofurky, Sweet Earth Natural Foods, and Field Roast, just to name a few. In other words, there's no need to ever ask "What do vegans eat?" It's simpler to question what vegans *don't* eat, as the list is much shorter! You may find it easiest to spend some weeks eating a vegetarian diet while gradually omitting eggs, dairy, and other animal products. Others prefer going "cold turkey." There's no right or wrong way to go vegan, but you'll need a little help along the way. No matter if you are a seasoned cooking pro or more apt to take-out meals, switching to a vegan diet has never been easier!

Wherever you're coming from, this planner will be your mentor at every step. But first, why is the vegan diet and lifestyle so important?

Why Vegan?

Chances are you've already put some thought into why you want to change your diet (and your life!) by going vegan. But before you even start trying to figure out what's for dinner tonight, take a moment to think about your goals. Why do you want to go vegan? What is your personal motivation? Personal health? Animal welfare? Environmentalism?

For many, personal health is a strong motivator to switch to a vegan diet. Many people of all ages report having more energy, enjoying clearer skin, and needing less sleep when following a healthy, plant-based vegan diet. Changing to a vegan diet can decrease your blood pressure in less than two months, and lower your cholesterol. A vegan diet is naturally cholesterol-free and is almost guaranteed to lower your cholesterol, often in as little as two weeks. Research from

People for the Ethical Treatment of Animals shows that a high intake of protein from plant sources can lower the risk of heart disease by 30 percent. But these benefits are just the tip of the iceberg.

From significantly reduced rates of hypertension, arterial hardening, stroke, type 2 diabetes, obesity, heart disease, and several types of cancer (prostate, colon, and breast cancer being the most well documented), eating vegan helps prevent the vast majority of life-threatening diseases that plague modernity. In fact, the World Health Organization (WHO) declared in 2015 that processed meat such as ham, bacon, and salami is a carcinogen. The American Dietetic Association affirms that a plant-based diet prevents many ailments, helps reverse some, and eases the symptoms of others. What's more, a study in the *Journal of Obesity-Related Metabolic Disorders* showed that vegans tend to have a lower body mass index (BMI) compared to non-vegans. Veganism isn't a bulletproof vest in protecting against these killers, but it is clearly an effective option. And it's not just your physical health that will benefit from veganism—your mental health will too. Studies in *Nutritional Neuroscience* show that vegans report less anxiety and stress as compared to omnivores.

Many professional athletes are opting for vegan foods to help them be at the top of their game. From tennis player Venus Williams to football player Colin Kaepernick, to race car driver Lewis Hamilton, just to name a few, more and more athletes are saying "no thanks!" to meat and dairy. Not only does veganism improve energy, it also improves recovery time. For instance, research published in *Clinical Cardiology* showed that eating vegan foods for just four weeks reduced inflammation by 29 percent.

In addition to the numerous health benefits of vegan foods, many are turning to plants due to increasing concerns over animal suffering. Gone are the days of Old MacDonald's happily mooing dairy cows and clucking chickens. Today's cows are relentlessly milked by machines, not cheery, freckle-faced farmers in overalls, and chickens rarely roam free in the fresh country air. Eggs today come from hens that are tightly packed into filthy cages, stacked floor to ceiling in huge warehouses. Under these circumstances, deaths from dehydration and suffocation are common. To avoid pecking conflicts, baby chicks have their beaks sliced off at birth. Dairy-producing cows must be kept constantly pregnant in order to lactate and produce milk, which is sucked out of them by powerful machines, and their offspring are regularly taken from them and sold to slaughterhouses as veal calves. When you research the treatment of animals by many meat manufacturers, it's no wonder that more and more people are opting for plant-based alternatives.

Modern food production is no friend to animals, your health, or the environment. Animal agriculture is responsible for more greenhouse gas emissions than all of the world's transportation systems *combined*. Raising animals for food also requires immense amounts of land, food, energy, and water, and with the world's populations set to reach 9.8 billion by just 2050, a more sustainable food system is needed. The United Nations has declared the impact of meat production to be "the world's most urgent problem" and recommends a shift toward plant-based foods. Animal agriculture is also the leading cause of animal extinction, ocean dead zones, and water pollution. One simply can't call herself an environmentalist while still consuming animal products.

VEGAN HEALTH AND NUTRITION

To reap the benefits of veganism, you need to eat wholesome, plant-based foods. After all, French fries and potato chips are animal-free, but that doesn't make them nutritious. When it comes to vegan nutrition, variety is key.

Essential Vitamins and Minerals

With a healthy vegan lifestyle, you'll likely find that your intake of many essential nutrients actually increases, rather than decreases, but it's still a good idea to make sure you're getting enough protein, iron, zinc, iodine, calcium, and vitamin D. The Dietary Guidelines for Americans (2015–2020) has started to shift from individual nutrients to healthy patterns. Towards that end, DGA established a Healthy Vegetarian Eating Pattern that's also relevant for vegans. This pattern specifies eating 2½ cups of vegetables and 2 cups of fruit per day with vegetable choices further broken down:

- 1½ cups dark green per week
- 5½ cups red and orange per week
- 3 cups legumes per week
- 5 cups starchy per week
- 4 cup other per week

This pattern includes extra legumes as a plant source for protein.

One important nutrient to be aware of is vitamin B_{12}, as it cannot reliably be obtained from vegan foods. Deficiencies of this important nutrient are admittedly rare, but long-term vegans and pregnant and breastfeeding women, in particular, need a reliable source. Because the body needs very little B_{12} and it can be stored for years, some people claim an extra supplement is not needed. The bottom line, according to most experts, is that when it comes to B_{12}, it's best for long-term vegans

to take a supplement. Better safe than sorry. Many of the recipes in this planner include a vegan food supplement called nutritional yeast, which is fortified with B_{12}, as are many plant-based milks (such as almond, cashew, soy, and oat milks) and veggie burger brands, so you may want to include these foods in your diet regularly.

You'll also want to be mindful of your iodine intake, which is simple to do when using iodized salt or sea vegetables (such as edible seaweed); iodine is key for a healthy thyroid gland!

Proteins

Despite a national obsession with protein, the truth is, most Americans eat much more than recommended, and deficiency in vegans is rare. Severe protein deficiency, called *kwashiorkor*, is a very serious problem sadly endemic in developing nations such as Haiti and parts of Africa, particularly among growing children. But it's virtually unseen in developed Western countries, even among vegans.

Plants have protein too, so most vegans meet their daily requirement of protein with ease. Just 1 cup of tofu, for example, contains 18 grams of protein, which is nearly half the USDA daily recommended amount for women. As a vegan, most of your protein will come from tofu, meat substitutes, beans, and lentils, but also whole grains, brown rice, nut butters, plant-based milks, and once again, those dark leafy greens. Quinoa, in particular, is the queen of whole grains when it comes to protein, with 8 grams per cup, cooked. What's more, the Beyond Burger by plant-based company Beyond Meat is the first plant-based burger to cook and taste just like a beef burger and boasts *20 grams* of protein per serving. Similarly, the Beyond Sausage, also made by plant-based company Beyond Meat, offers *16 grams* of protein per serving. Don't rely on just one source of protein, but eat a variety of nuts, beans, legumes, and lentils throughout the week.

Even as a new vegan, you don't really need to worry, as you'll probably consume more than enough protein without even thinking about it, but, as with other nutrients, make sure you're obtaining protein from more than one type of food and not just from beans or tofu alone, for example. In the words of the Academy of Nutrition and Dietetics' 2016 position paper on vegetarian diets, "Vegetarian, including vegan, diets typically meet or exceed recommended protein intakes when caloric intakes are adequate."

Fruits and Vegetables

Plan to get a wide variety within each food group. Broccoli is wonderfully nutritious, but you'll need to eat more vegetables than just broccoli in order to maintain a healthy and well-rounded diet. If you ate broccoli on Monday, try cauliflower on Tuesday and green beans on Wednesday.

Need a convenient way to remember to vary your veggies? Remember this: *Eat the rainbow*! Think of the colors of each fruit and vegetable—red strawberries, orange bell peppers, yellow squash, green romaine, blue blueberries, and purple eggplant—and rotate each color from time to time into your meals. It may be oversimplifying what nutritionists surely spent years studying, but "eat the rainbow" is an easy way to remember that each color found in nature provides a different nutrient, and for a healthy variety of nutrients, an array of colors is best!

In addition, every day should include at least one serving of fresh, raw fruits or vegetables, such as raw veggies dipped in hummus or dressing, a green salad, or even just an apple. The more fresh, raw, uncooked fruits and veggies you can include regularly, the better, and most days you'll easily get several servings rather than just one. But on busy days or when getting into new habits, it's easy to forget. Habitually eating fresh fruit first thing in the morning or making fruit the first snack you reach for is a good way to ensure you get fresh veggies and fruits every day. At the end of the day, ask yourself if you've had at least one serving of fresh, raw produce that day.

No matter what else you're eating, include several servings of green, leafy vegetables a week for optimum nutrition. There's just no substitute for fresh, raw, leafy greens, which are the most nutrient-dense foods on the planet. And finally, because it bears repeating, when planning your own vegan menus, don't forget that a healthy vegan diet requires a reliable source of vitamin B_{12}, preferably more than one.

Grains

Grains are one of your body's sources of energy. The key with any healthy lifestyle is to eat a variety of whole grains (such as brown rice, popcorn, hulled barley, quinoa, amaranth, millet, steel-cut oats, farro, sorghum, and whole wheat bread). Whole grains are chock full of nutrients including protein, fiber, B vitamins, trace minerals (iron, zinc, copper, magnesium), and antioxidants. Eating whole grains provides many health benefits, such as a lower risk of diabetes, heart disease, and high blood pressure.

Rice, for instance, is a versatile food that is easy to include into your diet. Two popular types of whole grain rice are "long grain" and "short grain" brown rice, with short grain tending to have a chewier texture. Finding whole grain alternatives to any refined grains in your diet is a simple way to add whole grains to your lifestyle.

Calcium

Calcium is an important part of any diet, mainly to keep bones and teeth strong but also to assist in certain metabolic functions. The Institute of Medicine in the United States sets the recommendation for calcium to be 1,300mg for people aged nine to eighteen, 1,000mg for adults, and 1,200mg for women over fifty and men over seventy. Green leafy vegetables are a great source of calcium. Non-vegans get the majority of their calcium from dairy sources, but vegans usually turn to dark, leafy green vegetables (such as broccoli and kale), calcium-set tofu, molasses, kale, broccoli, black beans, some legumes, and fortified nondairy milks. High-oxalate choices like spinach, beet greens, and Swiss chard have low absorption rates of their calcium content. Low-oxalate vegetables such as broccoli, collards, okra, kale, turnip greens, Chinese cabbage, or bok choy have higher absorption rates, meaning that your body can more easily access the calcium in them.

For comparison, 1 cup of calcium-fortified, unsweetened soy milk contains 300mg of calcium, while 1 cup of whole milk has 276mg of calcium. Half a cup of tofu (with calcium sulfate listed on the ingredients) has 430mg of calcium.

Calcium is important for bone health, but it's also important to consider vitamin D and exercise. With a well-planned vegan diet, as well as ample exercise, you can ensure good bone health.

SHOPPING FOR VEGAN FOODS

Health food stores and gourmet grocers stock plenty of vegan specialty goods, but these days most regular chain supermarkets also carry mock meats and dairy substitutes. Even retailers such as Target and Walmart carry vegan items! Some stores have a separate "natural foods" aisle, while others stock the meat alternatives with traditional meat. Most health food stores and co-ops are happy to place special orders, so don't be afraid to ask if there's something you'd like them to carry. Take a leisurely walk up and down each aisle of your grocery store and look for vegan foods that you've never tried before. The ethnic food section hides a wonderful array of vegan foods. You can usually find tahini, curry pastes, sauces, and several kinds of quick-cooking noodles. Take a careful look at the frozen foods aisle, and you're likely to find much more than just frozen veggie burgers. Frozen convenience foods may not be the healthiest option, but they're great in a pinch. Keep an eye out for delicious meat-free bowls from companies like Kashi, Gardein, and Sweet Earth Foods, not to mention dairy-free mac and cheese. Even if you prefer cooking most of your meals fresh, just knowing that alternatives are available if you need them can be comforting.

Seek out ethnic and import grocers for hidden vegan treasures, and if you're lucky, for basics at about a third the cost of other places. Miso, tempeh, and tofu, for example, are a bargain at Asian grocery stores. You can also find affordable canned jackfruit in Asian grocery stores, a tasty meat substitute. Besides just the deals, it's worth the extra trip to an Asian grocery to browse the mind-boggling options of exotic mock meat products you'll find there, from mock duck to vegetarian "shrimps" and "scallops." Kosher groceries stock enough dairy substitutes to fill a vegan's dreams, and Middle Eastern and Mexican grocers supply a bounty of ingredients, sauces, and spices to expand your palate.

Experimenting with all these new foods and flavors is part of the fun of going vegan, but of course, each time you buy a new product, you'll have to take a close look to make sure that it's actually animal-free. Getting in the habit of reading the ingredients list and nutritional data on the foods is quick and easy. Common animal products such as eggs, dairy, and fish are also allergens and are identified last, usually in bold font. And, as someone trying to improve their health, you may want to avoid a few other things as well. For example, it's better to leave the high-fructose corn syrup and all the highly processed and packaged foods it's in on the shelf, along with monosodium glutamate (MSG), even though these are both technically vegan. Partially hydrogenated oils are sometimes found in vegan foods, particularly in vegan dairy substitute products, though manufacturers should be moving away from them, thanks to the FDA determining that they are "not generally recognized as safe."

You may be concerned that all this grocery shopping for new ingredients will really add up and break the bank, but the truth is that the foundation of a healthy vegan lifestyle is based on some of the cheapest foods on the planet. Have you seen the price of cheese lately? It's not cheap! Sure, you need to buy a few spices to get started, but with a little planning and bulk shopping, in the long run, you're more likely to see your grocery bill go down, rather than up.

Beans are fairly affordable when canned, but they're a bargain when prepared fresh. Lentils are even cheaper and easier to cook than dried beans. Whole grains purchased in bulk are usually less than a couple of dollars a pound, and cornmeal for making polenta is even less. If you're on a budget, opt for cheaper meat substitutes, such as TVP (textured vegetable protein) and homemade seitan and tofu dishes rather than store-bought seitan, and use dairy substitutes

sparingly. Stretch more expensive meals or ingredients by adding a can of beans or tomatoes to whatever you're preparing, and serve with an inexpensive filler, such as rice. While not necessarily full of nutrients, pasta and rice noodles are also a bargain. Knowing the price and shopping around can help, if you've got options. For example, fresh greens may be a bargain at your local farmer's market, while apples are cheaper at your regular supermarket.

GOING VEGAN: WHERE TO START?

Common advice when going vegan is to eliminate red meats followed by white meats, and then spend some time eating just fish or a vegetarian diet before eliminating eggs, dairy, and other trace ingredients. While this method intuitively seems like a good idea and indeed works for some people, it's also a little bit backward. Here's why: Dairy, and cheese in particular, is often the most difficult food to eliminate from your diet. This is a good argument for gradually eliminating it *first* rather than last, as it may take the longest to wean you off of it. In fact, according to Dr. Neal Barnard, author of *Breaking the Food Seduction* and the president of the Physicians Committee for Responsible Medicine, cheese is quite literally addictive, containing compounds called casomorphins that act on the brain much like other drugs with a mild opiate-like effect. No wonder it's so hard to give up! The less you eat these addicting foods, the less you want them, so reducing your cheese consumption *now* is a great first step toward veganism, even if you're not already vegetarian. (Need further motivation to stay away from cheese? Consider this: Cheese gets it smell from the same bacteria found in unwashed feet and body odor.)

If you've decided that you're motivated and disciplined enough to go "cold turkey" (or you just don't really care for milk and meat anyway), go for it! While quitting animal products cold turkey or doing a gradual elimination are both great transition methods, there is also a third way of going vegan that balances the two with a "middle path."

The "middle path" way to veganism recommends reducing your overall meat and dairy consumption while increasing consumption of plant-based foods. Think of this as a "pre-vegan" adjustment period. Take meat away from the center of your plate and put it on the side. Instead of a full steak, cook up a stir-fry with lots of vegetables and a bit of beef over whole grains. Making a pepperoni pizza? Use half the amount of pepperoni you'd normally use, and pile on extra vegetables or use a pepperoni alternative such as Lightlife's Smart Deli Pepperoni. Don't give anything up completely, unless you're ready. Simply reduce the quantity and portions of meat and dairy foods you eat while increasing your plant-based ingredients.

During this pre-vegan phase, eliminate or reduce whatever's easiest for you first, and you're not likely to miss it while you work on eliminating the other foods. For example, switch to plant-based milks such as soy, cashew, or almond milk instead of dairy when cooking and baking, and use vegan mayonnaise on sandwiches. If you're a coffee drinker, opt for plant-based creamers such as from So Delicious, Ripple, and Califia Farms. You'll barely even notice both of these changes, even if you're not quite ready to make the leap from turkey sandwiches to Tofurky slices. These are great steps to take in the week or two before you begin the meal plans set forth in this planner. The pre-vegan adjustment period will help ease you in to a delicious plant-based lifestyle!

Making the Leap

Whatever method you choose for going vegan—gradual elimination, cold turkey, or the middle path—there's no need to leave behind your favorite foods. Whether you love a greasy pizza covered in pepperoni, cheesy pasta dishes, or just a plain old grilled burger and fries, there's a way to make it vegan. When the same sauces and spices are used in preparation, just about anything can be a pretty good stand-in for meat, and the textures and flavors of most dairy dishes are easily replicated. To experiment with ways of making your favorite meals vegan, check the index of a few good vegan cookbooks, or try typing your favorite food into an online search engine along with the words *vegan* and *recipe*.

While you're easing yourself into your new vegan lifestyle, you'll need to experiment not just with new foods, but also with cooking more often at home and altering the selections you make when eating out. Use your pre-vegan time as a great excuse to have fun trying new restaurants and new vegan—or even mostly vegan—dishes. In other words, give yourself a taste of what's to come. Ask yourself if you can really taste the cheese on your vegetarian sub piled high with vegetables, and ponder just how much you would miss it.

Once you're comfortable with a slightly adjusted diet, it's time to take the next step of an honest effort at eliminating animal foods altogether. But you don't have to be perfect just yet. During these first few weeks, strive for persistence and forgiveness rather than perfection. Don't be too hard on yourself, and recognize that your experience may not be the same as what you anticipated. Close your ears to anyone who says it will be easy just as much as to anyone who tells you about how hard it will be. It won't be easy, and it won't be hard: It will be an experience that you will get through to the other side.

If you do break down and grab a hamburger one night, your goal is to respond with patience and persistence, no matter what your mind might be telling you. Your mind will let you excuse just about anything if you let it: "Well, it's all over, I may as well give up now," or "This is way too hard. I can't do this." Instead of taking this hard-line approach, allow yourself the slipup, recognizing that change takes time. Be patient and compassionate with yourself. A minor slipup or two doesn't need to prevent you from being successful in the long run unless you let it. Give yourself a break and resolve to keep going. It's much better to eat a hamburger today and keep trying than it is to give up and eat a hamburger every day! Besides, since so many people are emotional eaters, beating yourself up over a slipup may make you more stressed and frustrated, which may lead to the urge to indulge in even more non-vegan foods. Of course, just about anything you crave has a vegan version, so try indulging with comforting vegan substitutes instead!

If you find yourself struggling, allow yourself one meal or even one day a week to eat meat and dairy. Perhaps a Saturday or Sunday evening. Knowing you can have steak on Sunday will help you stick to your seitan throughout the week, and soon you'll find you don't need that Sunday steak after all. Popular food writer Mark Bittman follows a "Vegan Before 6:00" approach where he eats vegan until 6:00 p.m. When you do slip up, try not to respond with frustration and self-loathing, but with cognizance and mindfulness. Ask yourself how you felt physically and emotionally after eating whatever it was. Did it satisfy you? Was it really what you wanted? Keeping a food log will help you identify these things

and remember them for the next time you find yourself tempted. You have the rest of your life to eat vegan, and today is just one day!

When you're tempted, return to your original reasons for going vegan. Was it a video you saw online? Rewatch that video once or twice a week to keep it fresh in your mind. Surround yourself with reminders of your motivation, whether it's pictures of happy rescued farm animals or pictures of pristine rainforests threatened with destruction for cattle-grazing land. If you are switching to vegan foods for health reasons, remind yourself of the plethora of health benefits. This motivation will keep you successful with a vegan lifestyle.

Cravings and Changes: Be Prepared!

Although it's much easier to stick with a vegan lifestyle than just about any other way of eating, a small minority of people who are used to eating a heavier, meatier diet may find that they are struggling with hunger as a new vegan. Remember, veganism is not a calorie-restricting diet, so the solution, of course, is simple. If you are hungry, it means you aren't getting enough calories. Eat more! It's unlikely that you'll experience this, but if you do find yourself constantly hungry or losing too much weight, opt for heavier foods such as nuts, avocados, and meat substitutes, and fill up on fiber to help you feel full. Beans, lentils, and whole grains are a good source. Vegan foods tend to be lower in calories than non-vegan foods, which means you may need to eat larger meals than you may be accustomed to. For example, 3 ounces of lean cooked beef has more than 150 calories, while three ounces of firm tofu has only 70 calories. You could eat two servings of tofu and still be consuming fewer calories than the beef! If you're hungry, fill up your plate with more food.

Even though there's no reason to ever go hungry with a vegan lifestyle, you may find yourself longing for specific foods. What's the difference between hunger and a food craving? If you're truly hungry, you'll eat just about anything to fill that physical void. But when you're craving a particular food, you're not actually hungry. You are usually trying to fill an emotional void with a particular comforting taste. The easiest way to distinguish between the two is to ask yourself: "Would I want to eat an apple right now? Or a green salad?" If the answer is yes, then you're probably genuinely hungry. But if the answer is no, because all you really want is some ice cream or chocolate, then you're experiencing a food craving.

Cravings are a normal part of life, no matter what you eat! Dealing with them as a vegan may be as simple as finding a vegan substitute for whatever it is you're craving, or it may mean getting a bit creative. Go ahead and indulge in some vegan junk food from time to time, if that's really what you need in order to keep you on the healthy path in the long run. Ice cream, potato chips, cookies, and chocolate all have vegan versions that are readily available. Just make sure it's an occasional indulgence and not a daily habit.

Even though a craving may seem to be for a particular food, it may actually be for a particular flavor or texture. A craving for sweet and sour chicken, for example, is mostly about the tangy sauce rather than the chicken itself. Why not cook up a chicken substitute or even tofu or tempeh in the same familiar sauce? Taste works in combination with all of the other senses. The visual presentation, texture, and feel of the food in our mouth, the smell, and even the sound a food makes as we chew it changes how we perceive it to taste.

This is why it's so easy to make the switch to vegan foods. Take tofu scramble, for example. A good vegan scramble has tofu that is crumbled to resemble scrambled eggs, and it also has a bit of yellow coloring added to it with turmeric, curry powder, or nutritional yeast. Some recipes even call for black salt, which gives it an "eggy" smell. When you combine all of these elements, your brain (and body) are pleased. So try a few substitutes with an open mind, and make your transition just a little bit easier.

Fighting cravings is also possible. Some people find that chewing gum helps a craving pass. Another tip is to eat something completely different to get your mind off whatever your craving is. Craving salty cheese crackers? Eat some sweet fruit. Your mind will switch gears, soon forgetting about the salt, and enjoy the sweetness instead.

One of the best ways to prevent those pesky cravings is to stay hydrated. It's common knowledge that staying hydrated has a multitude of benefits for your health, and one of these benefits is to keep you feeling full. If you're feeling hungry yet you've eaten sufficient calories, it may not be food your body needs, but water. Though nutritionists disagree about the best amount to drink, 8 ounces, eight times a day, is a good goal, especially when trying to improve your health.

Bring a reusable water bottle with you wherever you go and be sure to keep it filled up. Keep a water bottle in the car, at your desk, and in your bedroom. Get in the habit of drinking a large glass of water first thing in the morning. It'll help wake you up and get your digestive system moving in the right direction to start the day. If you also drink a glass of water before each meal and snack, you're well on your way to meeting your hydration needs. Another idea is to fill up a pitcher of water with two quarts (a little less than two liters) of water and make sure that you drink it all throughout the day. If you're not used to drinking so much water, you may find for the first couple days that you need to urinate more frequently, but your body will soon adjust, and you'll be rewarded with more energy, better skin, enhanced digestion, and better overall health. Record each glass of water you drink in this planner to make sure you're on the right track.

As your body adjusts, you may experience a bit of bloating as a new vegan. Although it's not often talked about, there's also the possibility of a bit of extra gas. Not everyone experiences this, but it can certainly be discouraging if you do! You can prevent bloating and gas before they even happen by drinking plenty of water. If you're cooking beans from scratch, make sure they're fully cooked, and switch out the soaking water with fresh water before cooking. When using canned beans, draining and rinsing them well helps rid the beans of the sugars that produce gas. Another culprit may be too much processed meat substitutes or even too much plant-based milk. Try sticking to simpler meals with fewer mock meats and switching to almond milk until your body adjusts to your new lifestyle. Ease back into the offending foods slowly, with small portions to start.

But it might not even be the new foods that is causing gas! Many enthusiastic new vegans are eager to experience everything the world of vegan food has to offer and end up overeating, which can also lead to gas. Consider your portion sizes. Maybe it's just too much food for your body to digest. Avoid eating when you're not actually hungry, and try not to eat too late at night.

Too late? Already bloated or gassy? Your first plan of attack is to drink a couple of glasses of water, and after that, get moving! Even though you might feel like you're about to burst like a balloon, a bit of exercise gets everything moving through your digestive track quicker. Even just fifteen minutes of brisk walking will help jump-start your digestion.

STAYING VEGAN: A LONG-TERM LIFESTYLE CHANGE

As a vegan, your entire relationship to food will change. This is why going vegan is much, much easier than losing weight! More often than not, weight loss diets fail. Why? Because most diets rely on restricting food calories or carbohydrates, which requires mental strength and willpower that most of us just don't have. Dieters still want that chocolate cookie or fried chicken, and without the strength and willpower to resist, they give in to temptation. Going vegan is easier than any other diet not only because you don't need to restrict calories or carbohydrates but also because you don't have to rely on willpower. Weight loss diets fail in the long term because nothing actually changes. The desire for junk foods or to overeat is still there. As a vegan, you won't want that cookie anymore, and you certainly won't want that fried chicken (and if you do, you'll choose the vegan cookie and the fried seitan). No, you don't need to somehow cultivate the iron will and self-control of a Buddhist monk to control your desires for meat and dairy. The difference is, as a vegan, your desires will change. Instead of relying on willpower, you simply won't want to eat meat and dairy. So how do you get to the point where you honestly don't desire those non-vegan foods anymore?

Veganism is not just another diet; it's a long-term lifestyle change. So you'll be changing not just the food on your plate, but also your mind. By investing the effort in exploring a vegan lifestyle, you've already begun the process of self-change. If animal cruelty is more important to you than a hamburger, then you won't want that hamburger. If lowering your cholesterol is a goal of yours, then you won't want to eat meat. If you're concerned about your carbon footprint, then you'll avoid dairy products. Because you've picked up this planner to explore going vegan, your priorities and motivations have already begun to change. What you want to eat today is different from what you wanted to eat two weeks ago, and it will be different from what you want to eat two weeks from now too. It's not just your mind that changes, but also your physical sense of taste. This is certainly good news for new vegans!

The longer you're vegan, the easier it becomes because your taste buds will change over time. Ever noticed that the more you eat spicy foods, the more heat you can tolerate? If you've ever gone a month or more without having a sugary soda, you'll know that the first time you do, it tastes unbearably sweet! This is because your taste buds react differently and adapt to whatever it is that you feed them over time.

Whether or not you're a smoker, certain medications, and even your genetics all play a role in developing and changing your own personal sense of taste. And, whether or not you change your diet, it's natural for your sense of taste to adapt and change over time as you age. It may take one month or it may take six, but at some point, you'll look at a pile of melted cheese and think to yourself that it looks rubbery and smells like mold.

But even with an array of all the best vegan ice creams, chicken wings, and hot dogs, you may still experience some setbacks. That's why your personal support system will have a huge effect on your success. Here are a few ways to make things a little bit easier for you.

Living and Eating with Omnivores

When you tell people you're eating vegan, something magical happens: It seems that everyone you know turns into an amateur nutritionist! Be prepared for lots and lots of questions and advice from people who are simply curious or well-intentioned yet ill advised. Everyone from your closest family to strangers on the street will want to know where you get your protein from and why you don't drink cow's milk anymore. Usually, they'll then start telling you how much they love cheese and how they could never go vegan. Meanwhile, if you're trying to eat, your meal is getting cold.

There will be times when you're happy to chat and talk about how much you love plant-based meat alternatives, but when you're in a hurry or just plain hungry, you'd rather eat in peace and enjoy your meal without having to defend your every bite. Offering to have the conversation later, after you've eaten, is a polite way to respond. You might also refer people to a few of your favorite books about vegan nutrition, such as *The China Study* by T. Colin Campbell and *How Not to Die* by Dr. Michael Greger. But there's no substitute for learning as much as possible. The more you know about the ethical, environmental, and health issues behind a vegan lifestyle, the more comfortable and confident you'll feel when engaged in conversations—willingly or not—with others.

Keep in mind that no matter who says what, you don't need to defend yourself to people who are less than well-intentioned when engaging you in discussions about your new lifestyle. Taking an ethical stance is not always easy, but if you believe that you are doing the right thing for yourself and for the world, then it will be just a little bit easier. Who cares what everyone else thinks? You are making the transition to veganism for your health, the animals, and the environment, and that's what matters!

Holidays and special events can be especially difficult to navigate, even for people who have been vegan for years. With a little communication and planning in advance, there's no need for any awkwardness. When it comes to special meals like Thanksgiving or dinner parties, don't expect your host to accommodate you without a little effort on your part too. It's always your responsibility to make sure your dietary needs are met. Offer to bring a vegan dish (or two or three!) to share, or, if your host would like more help, share a few of your favorite recipes or substitution ideas. Food is always a central part of holidays and social engagements, but if the goal is to come together as friends and family, the food should be what helps—not hinders—special events.

For formal restaurant meals, try to take a look at the menu in advance whenever possible. Vegan restaurant directories such as *HappyCow* and *VegGuide* are great resources for finding vegan-friendly restaurants. Don't be afraid to politely ask the waitstaff to help accommodate you. Unless the menu says "no substitutions," substitute away! Hold the cheese and chicken on the pasta special and ask for extra vegetables. A smile and a thank-you go a long way when making requests with waitstaff or inquiring about ingredients and substitutions. Restaurant chains such as Carl's Jr., Del Taco, Chipotle, Mellow Mushroom, White Castle, Burger King, TGI Friday's, P.F. Chang's, and The Cheesecake Factory all offer vegan-friendly menu options. If there's *really* nothing you can eat already on the menu, many chefs are happy to create a meat-free meal upon request. An even better idea

is to call in advance to ask about your options as a vegan and to let them know you'll be requesting a vegan meal.

Sit-down catered events are a little bit trickier, as there may be nothing on the menu to choose from. In a pinch, try to take a server aside discreetly, let them know where you're sitting, and request a plate with whatever side dishes they've got. Many are the times vegans have been relegated to eating a plain baked potato and plain steamed broccoli at weddings, fundraisers, and corporate seminars around the country, but not anymore. Vegan foods are becoming more and more mainstream, with options everywhere you look.

But no matter where you're eating, either at home in your own kitchen or in a five-star restaurant, the only person who ultimately matters is you. As a new vegan, you'll have enough on your plate (pardon the pun) without worrying about what everyone else is concerned about! First and foremost, take good care of yourself.

Avoid Temptation

Out of sight, out of mind is certainly a truism. If you're surrounded by bacon-cooking roommates or family, it will be more difficult for you than if you're living alone or with supportive people who are along for the ride. If your family and friends are willing to compromise, why not ask them if they'd help you out by not eating meat in front of you? They can grab a burger for lunch while you're at work, but come dinner, it's teriyaki tempeh time with no complaints!

If your refrigerator is filled with tempting foods, distraction will help you out until your cravings subside. Keep yourself busy, out of the kitchen, and away from temptation. Try to keep your mind occupied with things other than food. Read a good magazine or browse the newspaper while sipping an almond milk latte at a local coffeehouse if the temptation is too great at home. Try a new yoga class to occupy your evenings, or go through your *Netflix* queue (if you're looking for recommended vegan documentaries, check out *Forks over Knives*, *Cowspiracy*, and *What the Health*, all of which are available with *Netflix* streaming).

It's a bit more difficult to control your environment outside of the home. Social situations can lead to pressure to eat just to feel normal. Until you feel comfortable as a vegan and are past temptation, consider avoiding group meals when possible. Instead of meeting up for lunch with someone who might not be supportive, meet at a café for coffee or tea. Bring a few of your own hors d'oeuvres to share at a party, so you'll be less tempted by other foods.

Another way to keep food out of sight and out of mind is to turn off the TV. It's full of advertisements for foods that are rarely healthy, much less vegan. When was the last time you saw a commercial for plant-based meats or fresh spinach on TV? Watch your favorite shows online or record them to watch later to avoid fast-food ads.

Find a Support Network

If you don't have support within your home, find it outside the home or make your own! If you're lucky enough to have friends who are already vegan, now's the time to let them know your plans to transition to a vegan lifestyle and ask them for advice. Even if it's just a casual acquaintance, most people who are already vegan will be happy to share their experience and a few encouraging tips with you. If you don't know anyone personally, look online to find other vegans in your community (such as on Meetup.com), or check the bulletin boards of your local co-op or health food store. Vegan organizations and environmental groups often host vegan potlucks or restaurant trips where you can get to know other vegans in your area who can mentor you along the way. What's more, *Instagram* and *Twitter* are full of vegan bloggers who are ready to provide inspiration, and maybe even answer your questions. Before you know it, you'll be the expert whom other new vegans are coming to for advice!

Educate Yourself

Whether or not you have a strong support network (but especially if you don't), educating yourself with the facts about a plant-based diet will help keep you motivated if times get tough. Read up as much as possible about veganism and vegan health, browse vegan cookbooks for ideas, download vegan podcasts, and become immersed in the vegan community. Many health food stores offer free or low-cost vegan cooking classes. Surrounding yourself (and your online world) with constant reminders will only help you even more.

WHY YOU NEED THIS PLANNER

Some well-meaning people stop consuming milk, eggs, and dairy, but end up eating nothing but French fries, chips and salsa, or next to nothing at all, then wonder why they feel tired all the time after trying out a lifestyle that is supposed to be so healthy! They blame it on veganism, with unfounded claims that they aren't getting enough protein, and then switch back to eating beef and cheese. Of course, it's not lack of protein that is getting these unhealthy vegans down; it's a complete lack of *all* nutrients. Usually they say they didn't know what to eat, or that they were hungry all the time. Once you know about the incredible amount of options that vegans have to choose from, that sounds absolutely silly, but it happens quite frequently.

And it's exactly why this planner will come in handy! Eating delicious, healthy vegan foods for just twelve weeks is more than achievable and won't feel overwhelming to someone who has never dabbled in veganism. Plus, as *Psychology Today* reports, it takes only sixty-six days to make or break a habit…and you'll have eighty-four days! The research also shows that if you miss a day or two, you don't have to start the process over again. Just keep going! After twelve weeks of healthy, calorie-friendly vegan meals included in this week, you'll ease into veganism with confidence.

The meal plans in this planner gradually introduce you to the wide variety of foods available to you on a vegan diet. You'll try simple meals such as vegetable marinara and meat-free burgers; traditional favorites from around the world, such as pad thai from Thailand and chana masala from India; and you'll get a taste of vegan staples such as seitan, tempeh, and dairy substitutes. The preparation techniques and ingredients vary from day to day, so you'll never get bored with your meals, and there's always something new to try. Instead of wondering what to eat while you adjust to a vegan diet, the meal plans will do all the work for you.

While following the meal plans, you won't have to worry about nutrition, either. Besides including plenty of fresh fruits and vegetables, each day's meals are planned with attention to adequate protein, calcium, iron, and zinc, and while you may want to take a vitamin B_{12} supplement as a vegan, you'll often get more than enough from the foods included. While the USDA recommends no more than 2,300 milligrams of sodium per day (depending on your gender, age, and activity levels), you'll often consume much less than this. Another bonus? You'll be getting more

than 30 grams of fiber almost every single day. Increased fiber consumption has a myriad of benefits, including maintaining a healthy weight, reduced risk of heart disease and colorectal cancer, lowered cholesterol, and regulated blood sugar.

HOW TO USE THIS PLANNER

Each day, the meal planner provides you with simple meals that are easily adaptable to a busy lifestyle. Whether you're a single student, a working parent with a family to feed, or somewhere in between, you'll find the recipes quick enough to prepare on a daily basis. Weekend breakfasts are a bit more indulgent, and lunches are always planned with busy mornings and transport to the office in mind. Hopefully you have access to a refrigerator and a microwave or toaster oven at work, and can reheat leftovers. Nearly all of the dinner meals can be prepared in less than thirty minutes.

The menu plans rely heavily on ingredients that are easily accessible and affordable to the majority of people year-round, but similar foods can be used. For example, the suggested fruits are usually apples, pineapple, or bananas, but the most important thing is not so much that you eat a banana or an apple per se, but rather that you eat at least one piece of fresh fruit. Pineapple is a great source of vitamin C, apples are high in fiber, and bananas are very filling, but there's no reason that tangerines, watermelon, mangoes, and pears can't be substituted for any of these.

When it comes to fruit, eat what you like. Just like the type of fruit is merely a suggestion, so is the quantity. Within reason, it's impossible to eat too much fresh raw fruit and vegetables! So, eat more fresh fruit each day, and snack on extra baby carrots and snap peas, if you'd like.

A word of caution, however, when selecting fresh fruits and vegetables. Anything that comes in a package and needs an ingredients list doesn't count as fresh raw fruit. The same goes for vegetables. Banana chips, for example, are no substitute for the real thing. Skeptical? Read the label on a bag of banana chips; you'll see that they're coated in oil, with added sugar and often added salt as well. If you must substitute for fresh produce, go for frozen fruits and vegetables over canned, which nearly always have preservatives or added sugars and salts.

Grains are fairly interchangeable in the meal plans, as well, though each type has their advantages. Quinoa is a favorite among vegans for its nutty taste and high protein content. Couscous is not technically a whole grain, so it's a bit lower in nutrients, but it cooks quickly. You might prefer brown rice or white rice, as they're most familiar, and you may find that you begin to love instant rice for its convenience. If you're getting tired of rice, most stir-fries and curries do just as well paired with noodles.

Recipes are provided for some ingredients that you may occasionally prefer to purchase premade, such as hummus, vegan pesto, and salsa. When substituting these (or when making any other substitutions, for that matter), take a look at the nutritional information to make sure that the store-bought versions are of similar nutritional quality to the ones provided in this planner. Keep the nutritional information of store-bought goods handy by recording it in the extra space provided in the next section, Vegan Pantry. You'll also find there the list of common vegan foods helpful for making any substitutions or for adding any extra snacks to your meal plan. A few minor substitutions here and there are just

fine, but you'll want to keep careful track of your nutritional intake for any larger or frequent substitutions to make sure you're getting plenty of nutrients.

As you gain more experience in creating vegan meals, you'll find ways to personalize basic meals. A basic hummus wrap, for example, could have grated vegan cheese, pickles, olives, or sprouts, if you like them, and a tofu scramble can always have extra mushrooms or hot sauce, or whatever vegetables you need to use up. You'll be able to track these variations using the next section, Vegan Pantry.

BEFORE YOU START

A week or so before you begin, start to prepare your kitchen. Gradually get rid of any unopened non-vegan foods or condiments by donating them to your local food pantry, and start stocking up on vegan pantry items. (See the next section: Vegan Pantry.) Gather up a few reusable storage containers for leftovers and for transporting food and snacks with you. Even if you are at home during the day and don't need to worry about bringing lunch into the office, there will inevitably be some times during the next twelve weeks when you'll need a meal or at least some snacks when you're out and about.

Get Ready...

The equipment and utensils needed in a vegan kitchen vary little from what any other home cook might need. A blender for making healthy fruit smoothies is essential, and a food processor is helpful for making sauces such as hummus and pesto. Rather than working up a sweat grating carrots, a food processor will do the trick in just ten seconds! It's definitely worth it if you're cooking for more than just one or two people. Quality chopping knives and a cutting board are standard for any cook, as are a large skillet or sauté pan, a stockpot for soups, and some oven basics, such as a casserole dish and a baking pan. With these few items, you'll be prepared to create almost all of the recipes in this planner. Though not an essential, a rice steamer (or an Instant Pot®) means one less pot on the stove to worry about. After adding liquid and just about any grain (not just rice), you can walk away without worry.

Get Set...

At the beginning of each week, take a few minutes to skim through the meal plans and make sure you understand the requirements for the days ahead.

Each day's meal plans provide three balanced meals and a healthy snack.

- The plans are designed with the caloric needs of the average American woman in mind and provide roughly **1,800** calories each day.
- Most men will need to increase the portion sizes of each meal in order to meet their caloric needs, about **2,400** or more on average.
- Smaller women or those hoping to reduce weight may want to reduce their intake to about **1,600** calories per day while maintaining a total fat intake of 20 to 35 percent of total calories, and keeping protein to about 10 to 35 percent.

The following chart uses **2,000** calories as an average.

NUTRITIONAL GUIDELINES: RECOMMENDED DAILY INTAKE	
Calories	2,000
Fat	78g
Protein	50g
Sodium	2,300mg
Fiber	28g
Carbohydrates	275g
Sugar	No daily value
Added sugars	50g
Zinc	11mg
Calcium	1,300mg
Iron	18mg
Vitamin D	20mcg
Vitamin B_{12}	2.4mcg

Individualized nutrient needs are complex calculations based on age, gender, activity level, and weight status and are best determined by using an online calculator or consulting with a registered dietitian who specializes in vegan nutrition.

Read each recipe and check the serving size carefully. If you're cooking for more than just one, make sure you have enough food to adjust your portion sizes as needed, while still having enough leftovers as required by the meal plans.

Go for Your Goals

Get ready for day one. Write your goals down for your first day eating vegan and set a timeline for your transition. Don't just think about your goals; actually *write them down.* Just the simple act of writing switches on the gears in your brain, preparing you to go from thought into action. Effective goals take a bit of thought and effort. They should be as specific and concrete as possible, with an actionable timeline. They should also be quantifiable, so that you can assess your progress. "Eat healthier" or even "go vegan" are not specific time-oriented goals. Define your intentions clearly, using positive, uplifting statements. Rather than "I won't eat eggs and cheese," try "Starting tomorrow, I will eat a plant-based diet every day for twelve weeks. I will keep a food log every day, and spend fifteen minutes at the end of every week reviewing my progress!" If you've decided to transition more slowly, be as specific as possible with your goals. Instead of "I will eat mostly vegan for two months and then go fully vegan on January 1," define your boundaries concretely. What does "mostly vegan" mean to you? Perhaps your goal is to eat two vegan meals a day, or to eat vegan Monday through Friday for two months. Be as specific as possible and keep your goals handy. Check in on your goals at least once a week to monitor your progress!

Have you written down your goals? Good. Let's keep going!

Some people find it helpful to make visual representations of their goals to keep nearby to help remind themselves and focus their mind on the target. This can be as simple as a picture of a happy pig living a peaceful life at an animal sanctuary (or an unhappy cow connected to a milking machine) taped to your refrigerator or framed next to your bed, or as comprehensive as a packed vision board.

Let's go over just one more thing.

Have you selected when day one is going to be? Pick your day, whether it's tomorrow or still a month away, and fully commit to it. Take the steps you need to be fully prepared by the time day one rolls around. Be confident that by the time you get to day one, you'll be ready. For convenience in using this planner, make day one a Monday, and spend the Sunday before getting ready for the coming week.

USING THE JOURNALING PAGES

By logging and journaling your meals, you'll be able to keep track of what you're eating, jot down notes to remember about foods you ate, and celebrate your progress becoming a vegan. You can also use it to help you on days when you feel old cravings pop up. For instance, if you're feeling down on day twenty-one, review your notes from a previous day when you were feeling fantastic. That amazing feeling of clarity will come back again soon. But the most important reason to log your meals is because *it works.*

In a now-famous study of American dieters by Kaiser Permanente, researchers discovered one simple key to dietary change.

All things being equal to a control group, people were more able to control their eating habits and lost more weight when they simply wrote down what they ate every day.

Just the act of tracking their food intake alone made people more consciously aware of what (and how much!) they were eating. The weight loss was marked. Amazingly, the journaling group lost twice as much weight as their non-journaling peers. When it comes to veganism, weight loss and caloric intake may not be the focus, but the tools are the same for changing your diet successfully. Journaling keeps you accountable to yourself and increases your mindfulness and awareness. How many times a week do you really eat cheese anyway? If you're at all like most people, chances are you haven't got a clue. That's where journaling comes in! After each day's meal suggestions and recipes, you'll find a blank journaling page with the following elements to help you track your progress and celebrate your success.

Today's Vegan Plate

By following the menus set forth in this planner, you'll be sure to obtain a wide variety of nutrients, foods, and exciting meals every day, with enough choices to keep the food interesting and to keep you engaged. Plus, there'll always be something new every week. But when you're ready to try making a few meal plans of your own, you can use the Today's Vegan Plate icon as a guide for what types of foods you should eat (vegetables, grains, and so on) and in what proportion (for example, more vegetables than protein).

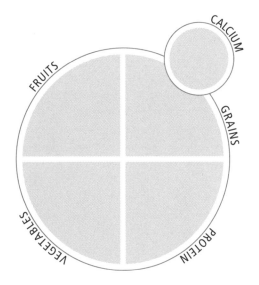

Each page in the daily journal includes Today's Vegan Plate graphic, on which you can check off the foods you're eating throughout the day. (This graphic is a variation on the USDA's MyPlate nutritional guidelines for healthy eating.) Throughout the day, add a checkmark to the correct food group on the plate icon when you eat a serving of something from that category. That way, you'll be able to see exactly which categories you have well covered and which you need to focus on more. Try to have your meals include more than one of the categories, and aim for a balance within all the groups every day.

Please note that the plate graphic should only be used as a visual guideline for your daily food intake and should not be used as medical advice. Your daily nutritional requirements may not always match up perfectly to the plate's sections. Please consult your doctor or a dietitian who has an understanding of vegan nutrition to set up personalized guidelines.

Today's Vegan Plate outlines five categories of foods and nutrients: grains (ideally, whole grains) or carbohydrates, proteins, vegetables, fruits, as well as calcium. Sounds easy, right? That's because it is! A simple vegetable stir-fry with tofu (protein) and brown rice (grain) would suit this plan perfectly, as would a bowl of whole grain cereal with fortified plant-based milk (calcium) and bananas (fruit). If you can't easily identify which of these groups a food belongs to, chances are it's been heavily processed with sodium or added sugars and is a food you should eat minimally.

Glasses of Water

Don't forget your recommended eight glasses of water a day! You can easily check off your water intake on the daily journal pages.

What I Ate

As you progress through the days, be diligent and honest about recording your meals and snacks. This planner provides daily journaling space for you to note the food you've eaten, how many servings you had, and its nutrition (calories, fat, carbohydrates, fiber, and protein). Much of the nutritional information you'll need can be found in the charts in this chapter—for any store-bought goods, check the nutritional label.

You may also find it helpful to note where you ate, or with whom, as well as any substitutions you made in food choices or food preparation. If you substituted an orange for a handful of carrots or used peanut oil instead of olive oil while cooking a meal, make sure that you list it even if it seems like it wouldn't make much of a difference. This will not only help jog your memory about a particular meal later on, but it can also help you identify eating patterns.

Thoughts about Today

Take a few moments to note how you feel periodically each day, or after a meal, in the Thoughts about Today section. Did a fruit smoothie make you feel wide awake and energized at the beginning of the day, or was it not filling enough, leaving you hungry by 10 a.m.? Some people find that too many meat alternatives feel heavy in their stomach and make them sluggish while other people like the satisfying "fullness" of a denser meal. Write these things down in the section titled "Thoughts about Today" so you can begin to see any emerging patterns to help you understand what's right for you.

Likewise, make sure you also note any slipups! If you find yourself scarfing down some cheese, write it down in this journaling section and note what else was going on that day to help figure out why you went for that cheese. Perhaps what you were really craving was salt, not salty cheese, and a bit of chips and salsa would have sufficed. Or perhaps you didn't get enough calories that day, and you were just looking for something to fill you up quick.

Week in Review

At the end of each week, review your feelings and your food choices on the Week in Review journaling page. What have you learned? What was the best or easiest part of the week and what did you find the most challenging? This journaling space gives you the opportunity to not only explore your feelings about the week and any challenges you faced, but also allows you to record your favorite memories and discoveries and new foods you'd like to try. Don't forget to celebrate and note your successes too. If you particularly loved a meal or a recipe, make a note. If you notice your skin getting remarkably clearer during Week 2, write it down, so you can remember it during Week 3 when you may experience temptation. If you try something new and particularly love it, write it down, and be proud of yourself! Keep a list of things to get excited about, such as vegan recipes you can't wait to try or restaurants you find that have great vegan options. You can also tally your weekly totals to see if you met the goals you'd set for yourself.

Welcome to the wonderful world of veganism! You're going to love it!

VEGAN PANTRY

Use this list as a guideline to help keep your cupboard and pantry well stocked, so that you always have the ingredients needed to whip up a quick and healthy meal, whether it's breakfast, lunch, or dinner.

CUPBOARD STAPLES

	Breakfast cereal
	Cocoa powder
	Couscous
	Egg substitute
	Flour
	Lentils
	Noodles
	Nutritional yeast
	Oatmeal or other whole grain cereal mix
	Pasta
	Quinoa or other whole grains
	White rice or brown rice

HANDY SNACKS TO HAVE ON HAND

	Nuts
	Granola
	Dried fruit
	Popcorn
	Soy yogurt

CONVENIENT CANNED GOODS

	Canned beans (black beans, chickpeas)
	Canned soups
	Canned tomatoes
	Vegetable broth
	Vegetarian baked beans
	Vegetarian chili

PERISHABLES

You shouldn't have to buy onions, garlic, and potatoes more than once a month. Vegetables for snacking include snow peas, baby carrots, and broccoli florets.

	Fresh fruit
	Garlic
	Hummus
	Onions
	Potatoes
	Tofu
	Vegetables for snacking

FREEZER GOODS

	Frozen fruit for smoothies
	Frozen vegetables
	Veggie burgers or other meat substitutes
	Ice for smoothies

REFRIGERATED STAPLES AND OTHER CONDIMENTS

Purchase the milk in aseptic boxes, if possible.

	Balsamic vinegar
	Barbecue sauce
	Dijon mustard
	Ketchup
	Maple syrup
	Olive oil
	Peanut, soy nut or almond butter
	Salad dressings
	Sesame oil
	Soy, almond, or cashew milk
	Soy sauce
	Tahini
	Vegan mayonnaise, such as Vegenaise
	Vegan margarine, such as Earth Balance

BREADS

These items last longer in the freezer.

	Bagels
	Flour or corn tortillas
	Pita bread
	Whole grain bread

GREEN SALAD FIXINGS

Lettuce greens include kale, romaine, baby spinach, rocket, and mixed greens.

	Artichoke hearts
	Bell peppers
	Canned corn
	Cranberries
	Croutons
	Cucumbers
	Kidney beans
	Lettuce greens
	Sunflower seeds
	Tomatoes
	Vegan bacon bits

SPICES

	Basil
	Bay leaves
	Black pepper (whole in a grinder is best)
	Cayenne pepper
	Chili powder
	Cumin
	Curry powder
	Garlic powder
	Onion powder
	Oregano
	Paprika
	Parsley
	Red pepper flakes
	Sea salt or kosher salt

VEGAN SUBSTITUTION CHART

Once you know a thing or two about some common vegan substitutes, veganizing your favorite recipes is easy. With a little know-how, you can find a reasonable stand-in for just about any ingredient you need, and you can make the same cookies, cakes, and muffins you've always enjoyed with egg and dairy substitutes. In fact, since most substitutes are lower in calories and fat and are occasionally cheaper, you'll wonder why you didn't make the switch sooner! Most larger grocery stores stock several vegan substitute products.

VEGAN SUBSTITUTION CHART		
INSTEAD OF THIS	**USE THIS**	**NOTES**
Butter	**Vegan margarine, soy margarine**	Vegan margarine works well in baked goods, sauces, and just about everything. Try Earth Balance or Miyoko's brands; vegan margarine comes in tubs, sticks, whipped, olive-oil based, soy-free, etc.
Milk	**Soy milk, almond milk, cashew, oat, hemp, or rice milk**	Rice milk is thinner and sweeter, with less fat. Stick with soy or almond for savory dishes and baking. Rice milk works best in smoothies and with breakfast cereals.
Creamer	**Soy creamer, coconut creamer**	Try Silk's Dairy-Free Soy Creamer, Califia Farms Dairy Free Better Half half-and-half creamer, or Coffee Mate's natural bliss Almond Milk Creamer.
Parmesan cheese	**Nutritional yeast, or Parmesan cheese substitute**	Try Parma! or Violife brands.
Egg	**Store-bought egg replacer, 1 T. flax meal mixed with 3 T. water, ¼ c. applesauce**	These egg substitutes work great in baked goods such as cookies, muffins, and cakes. For egg replacers, try Ener-G or Bob's Red Mill brand, or VeganEgg by Follow Your Heart.
Mayonnaise	**Store-bought vegan mayonnaise, homemade vegan mayonnaise, hummus, or pesto**	Vegan mayonnaise is quite tasty, but try expanding your horizons on sandwiches with different spreads, whether homemade or store-bought. For store-bought, try Follow Your Heart's Vegenaise.
Buttermilk	**1 T. lemon juice or vinegar mixed with 1 c. unsweetened soy milk**	It's not quite as thick, but the acidity of the lemon juice or vinegar provides tanginess similar to buttermilk.
Cheese	**Nondairy vegan cheese made from soy, rice, or almonds**	From Daiya, Field Roast, Follow Your Heart, Miyoko's, just to name a few, there is no shortage of dairy-free cheeses to choose from. Watch out for casein (milk protein) in other brands. Alternatives exist for everything from mozzarella to feta!
Chocolate	**Vegan chocolate**	Many chocolate bars and chocolate chips are dairy-free. Just take a quick skim of the ingredients list, or look for brands labeled as vegan.
Yogurt	**Dairy-free yogurt**	Try Silk, Daiya, or So Delicious brands. Check the dairy section of your grocery store.
Fish sauce	**Soy sauce with a squeeze of lime**	A common ingredient in Thai cuisine, vegan fish sauce is also available at some Asian grocers.
Oyster sauce	**Vegetarian oyster sauce**	Another ingredient common in Asian meals, the animal-free version is made from mushrooms and is standard in ethnic food aisles.
Honey	**Agave nectar**	Agave has a similar taste and consistency to honey, making it the perfect substitute.
Meat-based stocks, chicken broth	**Vegetable broth, vegetarian bouillon**	Avoid monosodium glutamate (MSG) in bouillon and powdered vegetable broth.

NUTRITIONAL INFORMATION FOR MORE THAN 300 COMMON VEGAN FOODS

Wondering what else you can eat as a vegan? Here are more than 300 common foods that you can easily include in a vegan diet. Though it never hurts to check the label of processed foods, all of the foods included here are free of animal additives. This list will come in handy at the grocery store when you're wondering what to eat, and when making substitutions or additions to the meal plans. You can also use this list when planning your own well-balanced vegan meals in the future. Just don't get too caught up in counting calories! Veganism is about discovering and enjoying new foods, not about restricting your calories.

Skim the list to find a few foods you already enjoy that are high in calcium, iron, and zinc, and make a note to include these nutrient-rich foods in your diet regularly. Use the extra space provided to note the nutritional data for store-bought foods or specific brands that you eat regularly.

BEVERAGES														
FOOD	SERVING SIZE	CALORIES	FAT	PROTEIN	SODIUM	FIBER	CARBO-HYDRATES	SUGAR	ZINC	CALCIUM	IRON	VITAMIN D	VITAMIN B12
Apple cider[1]	1 cup	2	0g	0g	34mg	0g	0.72g	0g	0.072mg	26mg	0.072mg	0mcg	0mcg
Carrot juice	1 cup	94	0.35g	2.2g	68mg	1.9g	22g	9.2g	0.42mg	57mg	1.1mg	0mcg	0mcg
Coconut water	1 cup	45	0.53g	2.4g	250mg	2.4g	9.5g	7.1g	0mg	57mg	0mg	0mcg	0mcg
Coffee	8 fl oz	5	0g	0g	5.3mg	0g	1.3g	0g	0mg	5.3mg	0mg	0mcg	0mcg
Cranberry juice	1 cup	144	0g	0g	5mg	0.3g	36g	4g	0mg	8mg	0.4mg	0mcg	0mcg
Fruit smoothies	berries, soy milk	166	5.2g	11g	135mg	4.3g	22g	9g	0mg	104mg	2.4mg	0mcg	2.4mcg
Grapefruit juice	1 cup	95	0.27g	2.4g	2.4mg	0g	22g	22g	0mg	22mg	0mg	0mcg	0mcg
Hot agave nectar-lemon water	1 cup	29	0g	0g	0.29mg	0g	8.3g	5.9g	0mg	2.2mg	0mg	0mcg	0mcg
Lemonade	1 cup	99	0g	0g	7mg	0.2g	26g	0g	0mg	7mg	0.4mg	0mcg	0mcg
Juice spritzer[2]	1 cup	28	0g	1g	38mg	0g	6g	5g	0mg	16mg	0mg	0mcg	0mcg
Orange juice[3]	1 cup	110	0g	2g	0mg	26g	22g	0g	350mg	0mg	0mg	0.408mcg	
Protein shake	1 oz of powder[5]	96	0.96g	23g	285mg	1.6g	2.1g	0g	1.1mg	50mg	4.1mg	0mcg	0mcg
Prune juice	½ cup	91	0g	0.78g	5.1mg	1.3g	22g	21g	0.27mg	15mg	1.5mg	0mcg	0mcg
Tea, chai	12 fl oz[6]	210	2.7g	4.2g	72mg	0.6g	43g	36g	0mg	210mg	0.9mg	0mcg	0mcg
Tea, green	1 cup	3	0g	0g	2.7mg	0g	0g	0g	0mg	0mg	0.13mg	0mcg	0mcg
Tea, black	1 cup	2	0g	0g	0mg	0g	0.71g	0g	0.024mg	0mg	0.024mg	0mcg	0mcg
Tomato juice[4]	1 cup	41	0.1g	1.8g	24.3mg	1g	10.3g	8.6g	0.4mg	24.3mg	1.0mg	0mcg	0mcg
Water	1 cup	0	0g	0g	0mg	0g	0g	0g	0mg	0mg	0mg	0mcg	0mcg

1. Powdered drink, 2. Club soda and ¼ cup of juice, 3. Fortified with calcium, 4. No salt added, 5. Mixed with water, 6. Starbucks

CONDIMENTS, SPREADS, AND SAUCES

FOOD	SERVING SIZE	CALORIES	FAT	PROTEIN	SODIUM	FIBER	CARBO-HYDRATES	SUGAR	ZINC	CALCIUM	IRON	VITAMIN D	VITAMIN B$_{12}$
Almond butter	1 tbsp	101	9.5g	2.4g	1.8mg	0.6g	3.4g	0g	0.5mg	43.2mg	0.6mg	0mcg	0mcg
Applesauce, unsweetened	1 cup	102	0.2g	0.4g	4.9mg	2.7g	27.5g	22.9g	0.1mg	9.8mg	0.6mg	0mcg	0mcg
Apricot preserves	1 tbsp	48	0g	0.2g	8mg	0g	13g	13g	0mg	4mg	0mg	0mcg	0mcg
Babaganoush	1 oz	80	8g	0g	0mg	1g	3g	0g	0mg	1.9mg	0mg	0mcg	0mcg
Barbecue sauce	2 tbsp	39	0.1g	0.17g	224mg	0.31g	8.9g	7.4g	0mg	5.1mg	0.21mg	0mcg	0mcg
Black bean dip	¼ cup	60	0g	4g	0mg	4g	12g	0g	0mg	0mg	0mg	0mcg	0mcg
Caramel	1 oz	108	2.3g	1.4g	69mg	0g	22g	19g	0mg	39mg	0mg	0mcg	0mcg
Cashew butter	2 tbsp	186	16g	6g	5mg	1g	9g	0g	2mg	14mg	2mg	0mcg	0mcg
Chocolate syrup	1 tbsp	54	0.22g	0.4g	14mg	0.5g	13g	9.6g	0.14mg	2.7mg	0.41mg	0mcg	0mcg
Cocktail sauce	1 oz	28	0g	0g	215mg	0g	6.5g	1.9g	0mg	0mg	0mg	0mcg	0mcg
Edamame hummus	1 tbsp	45	4g	1g	45mg	0.3g	1.5g	0g	0.19mg	11mg	0.62mg	0mcg	0mcg
Ginger dressing	2 tbsp	60	4.5g	0g	190mg	0g	5g	4g	0mg	0mg	0mg	0mcg	0mcg
Greek dressing	2 tbsp	100	11g	0g	310mg	0g	1g	2.3g	0mg	0mg	0mg	0mcg	0mcg
Guacamole	¼ cup	91	8.4g	1.1g	86mg	3.8g	4.9g	0.4g	0mg	10mg	0.3mg	0mcg	0mcg
Hummus	1 tbsp	25	1.4g	1.2g	56.8mg	0.9g	2.1g	0g	0.3mg	5.7mg	0.4mg	0mcg	0mcg
Italian dressing	2 tbsp	86	8.2g	0g	386mg	0g	2.9g	2.4g	0mg	2.1mg	0.29mg	0mcg	0mcg
Jam, sugar-free	1 tbsp	10	0g	0g	0mg	0g	5g	0g	0mg	0mg	0mg	0mcg	0mcg
Jelly (with real fruit)	1 tbsp	42	0g	0g	4mg	0g	10g	7.6g	0mg	0mg	0mg	0mcg	0mcg
Ketchup	1 tbsp	14.6	0g	0.3g	167mg	0g	3.8g	3.4g	0mg	2.7mg	0.1mg	0mcg	0mcg
Mango salsa	2 tbsp	20	0g	0g	130mg	0g	4g	4g	0mg	0mg	0mg	0mcg	0mcg
Mayonnaise	1 tbsp	37	3g	0g	96mg	0g	2g	1g	0mg	1mg	0mg	0mcg	0mcg
Mustard	1 tsp	5	0g	0g	5mg	0g	0g	0g	0mg	0mg	0mg	0mcg	0mcg
Nutritional yeast	16g	45	0.5g	8g	5mg	4g	5g	1g	3mg	0mg	0.7mg	0mcg	7.8mcg
Oil, olive	1 tsp	40	4.5g	0g	0.1mg	0g	0g	0g	0mg	0mg	0mg	0mcg	0mcg
Oil, peanut	1 tsp	39.8	4.5g	0g	0mg	0g	0g	0g	0mg	0mg	0mg	0mcg	0mcg
Oil, vegetable	1 tsp	38.8	4.5g	0g	0.1mg	0g	0g	0g	0mg	0mg	0mg	0mcg	0mcg
Olive tapenade	1 tbsp	30	2g	0g	160mg	0g	1g	0g	0mg	20mg	0.7mg	0mcg	0mcg
Orange marmalade	1 tbsp	50	0g	0g	11mg	0.2g	13g	12g	0mg	7.7mg	0mg	0mcg	0mcg
Peanut butter (natural)	1 tbsp	100	8g	5g	3mg	1g	3g	1g	0mg	0mg	0mg	0mcg	0mcg
Pesto	1 oz	130	13g	1g	240mg	0g	1g	0g	0mg	30mg	0mg	0mcg	0mcg
Raspberry vinaigrette	2 tbsp	40	1g	0g	60mg	0g	8g	6g	0mg	0mg	0mg	0mcg	0mcg
Salsa	¼ cup	15	0.21g	0.72g	320mg	0.55g	2.7g	1.9g	0mg	12mg	0.091mg	0mcg	0mcg
Soy sauce	1 tsp	3.6	0g	0.6g	335mg	0g	0.3g	0.1g	0mg	1.2mg	0.1mg	0mcg	0mcg
Sunflower seed butter	2 tbsp	185	15g	6g	166mg	0g	9g	0g	2mg	30mg	2mg	0mcg	0mcg
Tahini	1 tbsp	89.2	8.1g	2.6g	17.3mg	1.4g	3.2g	0.1g	0.7mg	63.9mg	1.3mg	0mcg	0mcg
Tamari	1 tbsp	4	0g	0.65g	333mg	0g	0.36g	0.12g	0mg	1.2mg	0.12mg	0mcg	0mcg
Tomato sauce (no salt added)	1 cup	90	0.54g	2.4g	27mg	4.9g	17g	9.8g	0mg	34mg	0mg	12mcg	0mcg
Vegan mayonnaise	1 tbsp	35	3.5g	0g	65mg	0g	0g	0g	0mg	0mg	0mg	0mcg	0mcg
Vegetable broth	1 cup	15	0g	0g	940mg	0g	3g	2g	0mg	0mg	0mg	0mcg	0mcg
Vinegar, apple cider	2 tbsp	6	0g	0g	1.5mg	0g	0.3g	0g	0mg	2.1mg	0mg	0mcg	0mcg
Vinegar, balsamic	2 tbsp	30	0g	0g	0mg	0g	8g	8g	0mg	0mg	0mg	0mcg	0mcg
Vinegar, rice	1 tbsp	5	0g	0g	60mg	0g	1g	0g	0mg	0mg	0mg	0mcg	0mcg
Worcestershire sauce	1 tbsp	12	0g	0g	170mg	0g	3.3g	1.7g	0mg	19mg	0.87mg	0mcg	0mcg

DAIRY REPLACEMENTS

FOOD	SERVING SIZE	CALORIES	FAT	PROTEIN	SODIUM	FIBER	CARBO-HYDRATES	SUGAR	ZINC	CALCIUM	IRON	VITAMIN D	VITAMIN B_{12}
Apple butter	2 tbsp	40	0g	0g	0mg	2g	8g	8g	0mg	1.9mg	0mg	0mcg	0mcg
Almond milk, sweetened	1 cup	60	2.5g	1g	150mg	1g	8g	7g	1.5mg	450mg	0.7mg	0mcg	3mcg
Almond milk, unsweetened	1 cup	40	4g	1g	180mg	1g	2g	0g	0mg	450mg	0.85mg	0mcg	0mcg
Coconut yogurt	1 cup	150	6g	1g	0mg	2g	0g	0g	0mg	0mg	0mg	0mcg	0mcg
Hemp milk	1 cup	65.6	4.8	4g	0mg	0.8g	0.8g	0g	0mg	0mg	0mg	0mcg	0mcg
Rice milk	1 cup	120	2g	0.4g	86mg	0g	24g	0g	0mg	20mg	0.2mg	0mcg	0mcg
Soy hot chocolate	1 cup	100	2g	6g	95mg	1g	20g	15g	0.6mg	300mg	1.08mg	0 IU	3mcg
Soy milk	1 cup	90	4.5g	7g	29mg	2g	5g	1g	0mg	80mg	1.4mg	3mcg	0.36mg
Soy milk, chocolate	1 cup	120	2.5g	5g	140mg	3g	19g	16g	0.6mg	300mg	1.08mg	0mcg	3mcg
Soy yogurt	1 cup	140	2.5g	5g	20mg	0.5g	28g	19g	0mg	8mg	0mg	0mcg	0mcg
Tofu crumbles	¼ block	178	12g	15g	2mg	1g	5g	0g	2mg	421mg	3mg	0mcg	0mcg
Vegan cheese	1 slice	40	2g	1g	120mg	0g	5g	0g	0mg	200mg	0mg	0mcg	0mcg
Vegan cream cheese	2 tbsp	90	8g	2g	115mg	2g	3g	1g	0mg	20mg	0.36mg	0mcg	0mcg
Vegan feta cheese	1 oz	90	8g	0g	190mg	0g	3g	0g	0mg	0mg	0mg	0mcg	0.7mcg
Vegan sour cream	2 tbsp	28	1.9g	3g	85mg	0g	<1g	0g	0mg	0mg	0mg	0mcg	0mcg

FRUITS

FOOD	SERVING SIZE	CALORIES	FAT	PROTEIN	SODIUM	FIBER	CARBO-HYDRATES	SUGAR	ZINC	CALCIUM	IRON	VITAMIN D	VITAMIN B_{12}
Apple	1 small	77.5	0.3g	0.4g	1.5mg	3.6g	20.6g	15.5g	0.1mg	8.9mg	0.2mg	0mcg	0mcg
Apple chips	1 cup	129	6g	0.29g	27mg	2.7g	20g	17.9g	0mg	0mg	0.2mg	0mcg	0mcg
Apricots	1 cup, halved	74.4	0.6g	2.2g	1.6mg	3.1g	17.4g	14.3g	0.3mg	20.2mg	0.6mg	0mcg	0mcg
Apricots, dried	1 oz	67.5	0.1g	0.9g	2.8mg	2g	17.5g	15g	0.1mg	15.4mg	0.7mg	0mcg	0mcg
Apricots, freeze-dried	1 oz	72	0g	0g	0mg	2g	18g	14g	0mg	0mg	0mg	0mcg	0mcg
Avocado	1 oz	44.8	4.1g	0.6g	2mg	2g	2.4g	0.2g	0.2mg	3.4mg	0.2mg	0mcg	0mcg
Banana	1 small	89.9	0.3g	1.1g	1mg	2.6g	23.1g	12.4g	0.2mg	5.1mg	0.3mg	0mcg	0mcg
Banana chips	1 oz	145	9.4g	0.6g	1.7mg	2.2g	16.3g	9.9g	0.2mg	5mg	0.4mg	0mcg	0mcg
Blackberries	1 cup	62	0.64g	1.4g	1.4mg	7.2g	14g	7.2g	1.4mg	42mg	1.4mg	0mcg	0mcg
Blueberries	1 cup	84.4	0.5g	1.1g	1.5mg	3.6g	21.4g	14.7g	0.2mg	8.9mg	0.4mg	0mcg	0mcg
Blueberries, dried	¼ cup	140	0g	1g	0mg	4g	33g	17g	0mg	2mg	0mg	0mcg	0mcg
Cantaloupe melon	1 cup, balls	60.2	0.3g	1.5g	28.3mg	1.6g	15.6g	13.9g	0.3mg	15.9mg	0.4mg	0mcg	0mcg
Cherries	1 cup	86.9	0.3g	1.5g	0mg	2.9g	22.1g	17.7g	0.1mg	17.9mg	0.5mg	0mcg	0mcg
Cherries, dried	¼ cup	39	0g	1g	0mg	1g	9g	6g	0mg	7mg	0mg	0mcg	0mcg
Coconut	½ cup	136	13g	1.2g	7.7mg	3.5g	5.8g	2.3g	0.38mg	5.4mg	0.77mg	0mcg	0mcg
Cranberries	1 oz	86.2	0.4g	0g	0.8mg	1.6g	23.1g	18.2g	0mg	2.8mg	0.1mg	0mcg	0mcg
Cranberries, dried	1 oz	86.2	0.4g	0g	0.8mg	1.6g	23.1g	18.2g	0mg	2.8mg	0.1mg	0mcg	0mcg
Currants	1 cup	63	0.25g	1.1g	1.1mg	4.5g	16g	7.9g	0mg	37mg	1.1mg	0mcg	0mcg
Dates	1 date	66.5	0g	0.4g	0.2mg	1.6g	18g	16g	0.1mg	15.4mg	0.2mg	0mcg	0mcg
Figs	1 fruit	46	0.21g	0.63g	0.63mg	1.9g	12g	10g	0mg	22mg	0mg	0mcg	0mcg
Grapes	1 cup	61	0.3g	0.91g	1.8mg	0.91g	15g	15g	0mg	13mg	0mg	0mcg	0mcg

FOOD	SERVING SIZE	CALORIES	FAT	PROTEIN	SODIUM	FIBER	CARBO-HYDRATES	SUGAR	ZINC	CALCIUM	IRON	VITAMIN D	VITAMIN B$_{12}$
Grapefruit	1 large	107	0.37g	3.3g	0mg	3.3g	27g	23g	0mg	40mg	0mg	0mcg	0mcg
Honeydew melon	1 cup	64	0.2g	1.8g	32mg	1.8g	16g	14g	0mg	11mg	0mg	0mcg	0mcg
Kiwi	1 fruit	55	0.91g	0.91g	2.7mg	2.7g	14g	8.2g	0mg	31mg	0mg	0mcg	0mcg
Kumquats	4 fruits	54	0.75g	1.5g	7.5mg	5.3g	12g	6.8g	0mg	47mg	0.75mg	0mcg	0mcg
Lemon	1 lemon	11.7	0g	0.2g	0.5mg	0.2g	4.1g	1.1g	0mg	3.3mg	0mg	0mcg	0mcg
Lime	1 lime	11	0g	0.2g	0.9mg	0.2g	3.7g	0.7g	0mg	6.2mg	0mg	0mcg	0mcg
Lychee	1 cup	125	0.8g	1.6g	1.9mg	2.5g	31.4g	28.9g	0.1mg	9.5mg	0.6mg	0mcg	0mcg
Mango	1 cup	107	0.36g	1.6g	3.3mg	3.3g	28g	25g	0mg	16mg	0mg	0mcg	0mcg
Oranges	1 large	87	0.21g	1.9g	0mg	3.7g	22g	17g	0mg	74mg	0mg	0mcg	0mcg
Papaya	1 cup	55	0g	1g	4mg	3g	14g	8g	0mg	34mg	0mg	0mcg	0mcg
Passion fruit	1 fruit	17.5	0.1g	0.4g	5mg	1.9g	4.2g	2g	0mg	2.2mg	0.3mg	0mcg	0mcg
Peaches	1 fruit	61	0.35g	1.6g	0mg	3.1g	16g	13g	0mg	9.4mg	0mg	0mcg	0mcg
Peaches, freeze-dried	1 oz	97	0g	1g	11mg	1g	25g	17g	0mg	30mg	0mg	0mcg	0mcg
Pears	1 fruit	121	0.23g	0g	2.1mg	6.3g	31g	21g	0mg	19mg	0mg	0mcg	0mcg
Pears, freeze-dried	½ oz	40	0g	0g	4mg	1g	8g	7g	0mg	0mg	0.85mg	0mcg	0mcg
Pears, poached	1 fruit	185	1g	11g	0mg	4g	45g	21g	0mg	19mg	0mg	0mcg	0mcg
Persimmon	1 fruit	32	0.1g	0.2g	0.25mg	0g	8.4g	0g	0mg	6.8mg	0.63mg	0mcg	0mcg
Pineapple	1 cup	82.5	0.2g	0.9g	1.7mg	2.3g	21.6g	16.3g	0.2mg	21.5mg	0.5mg	0mcg	0mcg
Plantain	½ cup	90	0.25g	0.74g	2.9mg	1.5g	24g	11g	0mg	2.2mg	0.74mg	0mcg	0mcg
Plums	1 fruit	31	0.22g	0.67g	0mg	0.67g	7.3g	6.7g	0mg	4mg	0mg	0mcg	0mcg
Pomegranate	1 fruit	105	0.51g	1.5g	4.6mg	1.5g	26g	26g	0mg	4.6mg	0mg	0mcg	0mcg
Prunes, stewed	¼ cup	78	0.15g	0.69g	1.4mg	0g	21g	0g	0mg	17mg	0.69mg	0mcg	0mcg
Quince	1 fruit	52	0.1g	0g	3.6mg	1.8g	14g	0g	0mg	10mg	0.91mg	0mcg	0mcg
Raisins	1 oz	84.5	0.1g	0.9g	3.1mg	1g	22.4g	16.7g	0.1mg	14.1mg	0.5mg	0mcg	0mcg
Raspberries	1 cup	64	1.2g	1.2g	1.2mg	8.6g	15g	4.9g	0mg	31mg	1.2mg	0mcg	0mcg
Rhubarb	1 cup	26	0.27g	1.2g	4.9mg	2.4g	6.1g	1.2g	0mg	105mg	0mg	0mcg	0mcg
Strawberries	1 cup	48.6	0.5g	1g	1.5mg	3g	11.7g	7.4g	0.2mg	24.3mg	0.6mg	0mcg	0mcg
Strawberries, freeze-dried	1 oz	62	0g	0g	0mg	6g	16g	10g	0mg	0mg	0mg	0mcg	0mcg
Tangerine	1 cup	103	0.6g	1.6g	3.9mg	3.5g	26g	20.6g	0.1mg	72.2mg	0.3mg	0mcg	0mcg
Watermelon	1 cup	46	0.17g	1.5g	1.5mg	0g	12g	9.2g	0mg	11mg	0mg	0mcg	0mcg

GRAINS

FOOD	SERVING SIZE	CALORIES	FAT	PROTEIN	SODIUM	FIBER	CARBO-HYDRATES	SUGAR	ZINC	CALCIUM	IRON	VITAMIN D	VITAMIN B12
Amaranth	¼ cup	182	3.2g	7g	10mg	4.5g	32g	0g	1.5mg	75mg	3.7mg	0mcg	0mcg
Bagel, plain	1 small bagel[3]	146	0.9g	5.7g	255mg	1.3g	29g	2.9g	1.1mg	50.7mg	3.4mg	0mcg	0mcg
Bagel, whole wheat	1 small bagel[3]	262	1.6g	10.7g	461mg	4.3g	51g	6.4g	1.2mg	21mg	2.9mg	0mcg	0mcg
Barley, flakes[1]	1 cup	141	1.1g	4g	186mg	3.4g	32g	6.8g	1.6mg	15mg	11mg	27mcg	2mcg
Barley, pearled	¼ cup	176	0.56g	5g	4.5mg	8g	39g	0.5g	1mg	15mg	1.5mg	0mcg	0mcg
Bulgur	1 cup	151	0.4g	5.5g	9.1mg	9.1g	35g	0g	1.8mg	18mg	1.8mg	0mcg	0mcg
Buckwheat flour	¼ cup	101	0.9g	3.9g	3.3mg	3g	21g	0.9g	0.9mg	12mg	1.2mg	0mcg	0mcg
Buckwheat groats	1 cup	155	1g	5.7g	6.7mg	4.5g	34g	1.5g	1mg	12mg	1.3mg	0mcg	0mcg
Cornmeal	½ cup	251	1.4g	5.5g	2.1mg	4.8g	53g	0.68g	0.68mg	3.4mg	2.7mg	0mcg	0mcg
Couscous	1 cup, cooked	175	0.17g	6.3g	7.8mg	1.6g	36g	0g	0mg	13mg	0mg	0mcg	0mcg
Couscous[2]	¼ cup	173	1.5g	7.5g	0mg	4.5g	36g	0.8g	0mg	20mg	1.82mg	0mcg	0mcg
Cream of wheat	1 cup	31.5	0.6g	4.4g	364mg	1.4g	31.5g	0.2g	0.4mg	154mg	12mg	0mcg	0mcg
English muffin	1 muffin	140	1.1g	5.4g	248mg	1.5g	27.4g	1.8g	0.7mg	102mg	2.4mg	0mcg	0mcg
Granola	⅓ cup	194	10g	5.2g	71.1mg	3.7g	23.2g	7.7g	1.2mg	36.7mg	1.4mg	0mcg	0mcg
Grits	1 cup	143	0.5g	3.4g	540mg	0.7g	31.1g	0.2g	0.2mg	7.3mg	1.5mg	0mcg	0mcg
Millet	¼ cup	189	2g	5.5g	2.5mg	4.5g	37g	0g	1mg	4mg	1.5mg	0mcg	0mcg
Oat bran	¼ cup	56	2g	4g	1mg	3g	15g	0g	1mg	13mg	1mg	0mcg	0mcg
Oat groats	¼ cup	110	2.5g	7g	0mg	4g	27g	1g	0mg	20mg	0mg	0mcg	0mcg
Oats, steel-cut	½ cup	152	2.7g	6.6g	0.78mg	4.3g	26g	0g	1.6mg	21mg	2mg	0mcg	0mcg
Pita	1 pita[4]	165	0.7g	5.5g	322mg	1.3g	33.4g	0.8g	0.5mg	51.6mg	1.6mg	0mcg	0mcg
Polenta	½ cup	252	1.1g	6g	2.1mg	5g	54g	0.44g	0.5mg	3.4mg	2.8mg	0mcg	0mcg
Quinoa	1 cup	222	3.6g	8.1g	13mg	5.2g	39.4g	0g	2mg	31.5mg	2.8mg	0mcg	0mcg
Rice, brown	1 cup	216	1.8g	5g	9.8mg	3.5g	44.8g	0.7g	1.2mg	19.5mg	0.8mg	0mcg	0mcg
Rice cake	1 oz	110	1.2g	2g	19.9mg	1.2g	22.7g	0.2g	0.8mg	3.1mg	0.4mg	0mcg	0mcg
Rice noodles	1 cup	192	0.4g	1.6g	33.4mg	1.8g	43.8g	0g	0.4mg	7mg	0.2mg	0mcg	0mcg
Rice, white	1 cup	169	0.3g	3.5g	8.7mg	1.7g	36.7g	0.1g	0.7mg	3.5mg	0.2mg	0mcg	0mcg
Rye	¼ cup	146	1.3g	6.4g	2.5mg	6.4g	30g	0.42g	1.7mg	14mg	1.3mg	0mcg	0mcg
Spelt	1 cup cooked	246	1.6g	10g	9.7mg	7.6g	51g	0g	2.4mg	19.4mg	3.2mg	0mcg	0mcg
Spelt bread	1 slice	70	0g	3g	150mg	2g	16g	2g	0mg	0mg	0mg	0mcg	0mcg
Soba noodles	1 cup	113	0.1g	5.8g	68.4mg	0g	24.4g	0g	0.1mg	4.6mg	0.5mg	0mcg	0mcg
Taco shell, hard	1 shell[5]	58.2	2.6g	0.9g	48.6mg	0.6g	7.9g	0.2g	0.2mg	12.6mg	0.2mg	0mcg	0mcg
Teff	½ cup uncooked	354	2.3g	12.8g	11.5mg	7.7g	70g	1.8g	3.5mg	173mg	7mg	0mcg	0mcg
Tortilla, flour	medium, 8"	146	3.1	4.4g	249mg	0g	25.3g	0g	0mg	97.4mg	1mg	0mcg	0mcg
Tortilla, flour	large, 10"	296	8.5g	7.0g	662mg	2.8g	49.3g	2.8g	0mg	141mg	2.5mg	0mcg	0mcg
Triticale	¼ cup	161	1g	6.3g	2.4mg	0g	35g	0g	1.7mg	18mg	1.2mg	0mcg	0mcg
Panfried polenta	1 oz	101	1g	2.3g	9.8mg	2g	21.5g	0.2g	0.5mg	1.7mg	1mg	0mcg	0mcg
Pizza dough	2 oz	120	1.1g	4g	240mg	2g	24g	0g	0mg	0mg	0mg	0mcg	0mcg
Popcorn	1 cup	30.6	0.3g	1g	0.3mg	1.2g	6.2g	0g	0.3mg	0.8mg	0.2mg	0mcg	0mcg

1. Cereal, 2. Whole wheat, 3. 3" diameter, 4. 6½" diameter, 5. 5" diameter

GRAINS—CONTINUED

FOOD	SERVING SIZE	CALORIES	FAT	PROTEIN	SODIUM	FIBER	CARBO-HYDRATES	SUGAR	ZINC	CALCIUM	IRON	VITAMIN D	VITAMIN B12
Vegetable pasta	½ cup	76	0.57g	2.9g	3.4mg	0g	14g	0g	0.57mg	10mg	0.57mg	0mcg	0mcg
Wheat berries	½ cup	151	1g	6g	0mg	4g	29g	0g	5.6mg	15mg	7mg	0mcg	0mcg
Whole grain vegan bread	1 slice	69.1	1.1g	3.5g	110mg	1.9g	11.3g	1.7g	0.4g	26.6mg	0.7mg	0mcg	0mcg
Whole grain cereal (fortified)	¾ cup	100	0.5g	2g	190mg	2.7g	23.2g	5g	15mg	1,000mg	18mg	39.9mcg	6mcg
Whole wheat pasta	½ cup	100	1.7g	5g	308mg	2.5g	23g	0g	0.5mg	14mg	1.5mg	0mcg	0mcg

MEAT REPLACEMENTS

FOOD	SERVING SIZE	CALORIES	FAT	PROTEIN	SODIUM	FIBER	CARBO-HYDRATES	SUGAR	ZINC	CALCIUM	IRON	VITAMIN D	VITAMIN B12
Black bean burger	1 burger	264	1g	15g	391mg	9.7g	49g	1.4g	2.6mg	79mg	3.8mg	0mcg	0mcg
Falafel	1 patty	57	3g	2.3g	50mg	1g	5.4g	0g	0.26mg	9.2mg	0.58mg	0mcg	0mcg
Grilled chicken substitute[1]	3 oz	153	4g	23.5g	388mg	3.5g	5.9g	0g	0mg	47mg	3.1mg	0mcg	0mcg
Ground beef substitute[2]	½ cup	60	0.5g	13g	270mg	3g	6g	0g	0mg	60mg	1.8mg	0mcg	0mcg
Seitan	3 oz	90	1g	18g	380mg	1g	3g	0g	0mg	0mg	1mg	0mcg	0mcg
Tempeh	½ cup	161	9.2g	16g	7.5mg	0g	7.5g	0g	0.83mg	93mg	2.5mg	0mcg	0mcg
Tofu, baked	½ cup	88.2	5.3g	10.3g	15.1mg	1.1g	2.1g	0.8g	1mg	253mg	2mg	0mcg	0mcg
Vegan chicken	3 oz	120	5g	9g	210mg	4g	11g	0g	0mg	35mg	15mg	0mcg	0mcg
Vegan chicken patty burger	1 patty	140	5g	8g	590mg	2g	16g	1g	0mg	0mg	0mg	0mcg	0mcg
Veggie burger	1 patty	124	4.4g	11g	398mg	3.4g	10g	0.7g	0.9mg	95.2mg	1.7mg	0mcg	1.4mcg
Vegan sausage	1 patty	80	3g	10g	260mg	1g	3g	1g	0mg	3mg	1.44mg	0mcg	2.1mcg
Vegan pepperoni	13 slices	50	1g	9g	240mg	1g	2g	0g	0mg	0mg	0.36mg	0mcg	0mcg
Vegan hot dogs	1 link	80	2g	11g	390mg	3g	5g	0g	0mg	2mg	4mg	0mcg	0mcg

1. Beyond Meat, 2. Sautéed

NUTS AND SEEDS

FOOD	SERVING SIZE	CALORIES	FAT	PROTEIN	SODIUM	FIBER	CARBO-HYDRATES	SUGAR	ZINC	CALCIUM	IRON	VITAMIN D	VITAMIN B12
Almonds	1 oz	161	13.8g	5.9g	0.3mg	3.4g	6.1g	1.1g	0.9mg	73.9mg	1mg	0mcg	0mcg
Brazilian nuts	¼ cup	218	22g	4.75g	1mg	2.5g	4g	0.77g	1.35mg	53.25mg	0.8mg	0mcg	0mcg
Cashew	1 oz	155	12.3g	5.1g	3.4mg	0.9g	9.2g	1.7g	1.6mg	10.4mg	1.9mg	0mcg	0mcg
Chestnuts, roasted	½ cup	175	1.6g	2.1g	1.4mg	3.6g	38g	7.9g	0.71mg	21mg	0.71mg	0mcg	0mcg
Chia seed	½ oz	69	4.4g	2.2g	2.7mg	5.3g	6.2g	0g	0.49mg	89mg	0mg	0mcg	0mcg
Flaxseed	2 tbsp	104	8.2g	3.5g	5.9mg	5.3g	5.7g	0.39g	0.78mg	50mg	1.2mg	0mcg	0mcg
Hazelnuts	¼ cup	180	18g	4.3g	0mg	2.9g	4.9g	1.1g	0.57mg	33mg	1.4mg	0mcg	0mcg
Macadamia nuts	¼ cup	239	25g	3g	2mg	3g	5g	2g	0mg	28mg	1mg	0mcg	0mcg
Nuts, mixed	1 oz	172	15.7g	4.3g	85.7mg	1.5g	6.2g	1.2g	1.3mg	29.7mg	0.7mg	0mcg	0mcg

NUTS AND SEEDS—CONTINUED

FOOD	SERVING SIZE	CALORIES	FAT	PROTEIN	SODIUM	FIBER	CARBO-HYDRATES	SUGAR	ZINC	CALCIUM	IRON	VITAMIN D	VITAMIN B12
Peanuts, dry-roasted	1 oz	164	13.9g	6.6g	1.7mg	2.2g	6g	1.2g	0.9mg	15.1mg	0.6mg	0mcg	0mcg
Peanuts, oil-roasted	1 oz	168	14.7g	7.8g	89.6mg	2.6g	4.3g	1.2g	0.9mg	17.1mg	0.4mg	0mcg	0mcg
Pecans	1 oz	193	20.2g	2.6g	0mg	2.7g	3.9g	1.1g	1.3mg	19.6mg	0.7mg	0mcg	0mcg
Pine nuts	¼ cup	190	17g	8.3g	1.2mg	1.2g	4.8g	0g	0mg	8.3mg	3.6mg	0mcg	0mcg
Pistachios	¼ cup	170	13g	6.4g	0.3mg	3g	8.5g	2.4g	0.61mg	33mg	1.2mg	0mcg	0mcg
Pumpkin seeds	¼ cup	185	16g	8.6g	6.2mg	1.4g	6.2g	0.34g	2.4mg	15mg	5.1mg	0mcg	0mcg
Soy nuts	1 oz	126	6.1g	11.1g	0.6mg	2.3g	9.2g	0g	1.3mg	39.2mg	1.1mg	0mcg	0mcg
Sunflower seeds	¼ cup with hulls	65	5.7g	2.6g	0.34mg	1.3g	2.2g	0.34g	0.57mg	13mg	0.8mg	0mcg	0mcg
Walnuts	1 oz	185	18.4g	4.3g	0.6mg	1.9g	3.9g	0.7g	0.9mg	27.7mg	0.8mg	0mcg	0mcg

SPICES

FOOD	SERVING SIZE	CALORIES	FAT	PROTEIN	SODIUM	FIBER	CARBO-HYDRATES	SUGAR	ZINC	CALCIUM	IRON	VITAMIN D	VITAMIN B12
Basil	¼ cup	3	0.11g	0.32g	0.42mg	0.42g	0.42g	0g	0.11mg	16mg	0.32mg	0mcg	0mcg
Bay leaf	2 leaves	18	0.45g	0.45g	1.3mg	1.5g	4.3g	0g	0.23mg	47mg	2.4mg	0mcg	0mcg
Cayenne pepper	1 tsp	5.6	0.3g	0.2g	0.5mg	0.5g	1g	0.2g	0mg	2.6mg	0.1mg	0mcg	0mcg
Caraway seed	1 tbsp	22	0.98g	1.3g	1.1mg	2.5g	3.3g	0g	0.37mg	46mg	1.1mg	0mcg	0mcg
Chives	2 tbsp	2	0.061g	0.18g	0.18mg	0.18g	0.24g	0.12g	0.061mg	5.6mg	0.12mg	0mcg	0mcg
Cilantro	¼ cup	0.9	0g	0.1g	1.8mg	0.1g	0.1g	0g	0mg	2.7mg	0.1mg	0mcg	0mcg
Clove	1 tsp ground	7	0.44g	0.13g	5.4mg	0.76g	1.4g	0g	0.022mg	14mg	0.2mg	0mcg	0mcg
Cinnamon	1 tsp	6.2	0g	0.1g	0.2mg	1.3g	2g	0.1g	0mg	25.1mg	0.2mg	0mcg	0mcg
Cocoa powder	2 tbsp[1]	40	1g	2g	0mg	2g	6g	0g	0mg	0mg	3.6mg	0mcg	0mcg
Cumin	1 tsp	7	0.43g	0.35g	3.3mg	0.22g	0.86g	0g	0.098mg	18mg	1.3mg	0mcg	0mcg
Dill	¼ cup fresh	1	0.025g	0.068g	1.4mg	0.045g	0.16g	0g	0.023mg	4.7mg	0.16mg	0mcg	0mcg
Fennel seed	1 tbsp	20	0.88g	0.94g	5.2mg	2.4g	3.1g	0g	0.24mg	70mg	1.1mg	0mcg	0mcg
Garlic	1 tbsp	13	0.084g	0.51g	1.4mg	0.17g	2.8g	0.084g	0.084mg	15mg	0.17mg	0mcg	0mcg
Ginger root	1 tsp	5	0g	0.13g	0.81mg	0.13g	1.1g	0.13g	0mg	1mg	0.063mg	0mcg	0mcg
Horseradish	1 tbsp	7	0.15g	0.15g	47mg	0.45g	1.6g	1.2g	0.15mg	8.4mg	0mg	0mcg	0mcg
Lavender	1 tsp	0	0g	0g	0mg	0g	1g	0g	0mg	0mg	0mg	0mcg	0mcg
Marjoram	1 tsp dried	2	0g	0g	0mg	0g	0g	0g	0mg	11mg	0mg	0mcg	0mcg
Mint	2 tbsp	4.9	0.1g	0.4g	3.4mg	0.8g	0.9g	0g	0.1mg	22.4mg	1.3mg	0mcg	0mcg
Mustard seeds	1 tsp	18	1.1g	0.94g	0.19mg	0.56g	1.3g	0.26g	0.22mg	20mg	0.37mg	0mcg	0mcg
Paprika	1 tbsp	21	0.93g	1.1g	2.4mg	2.6g	4g	0.71g	0.29mg	13mg	1.7mg	0mcg	0mcg
Parsley	¼ cup	5	0g	0g	7.5mg	0g	1.3g	0g	0mg	18mg	1.3mg	0mcg	0mcg
Peppermint	1 tbsp	1	0.015g	0.06g	0.5mg	0.13g	0.24g	0g	0.018mg	3.9mg	0.081mg	0mcg	0mcg
Rosemary	1 tbsp fresh	2	0.1g	0.051g	0.44mg	0.24g	0.36g	0g	0.017mg	5.4mg	0.12mg	0mcg	0mcg
Tarragon	1 tsp dried	2	0.042g	0.14g	0.37mg	0.042g	0.3g	0g	0.024mg	6.8mg	0.19mg	0mcg	0mcg
Thyme	1 tbsp	2	0g	0.14g	0.22mg	0.34g	0.58g	0g	0.048mg	9.7mg	0.41mg	0mcg	0mcg
Turmeric	1 tsp	8	0.22g	0.18g	0.84mg	0.47g	1.4g	0g	0.089mg	4.1mg	0.91mg	0mcg	0mcg
Wasabi	1 tbsp	9	0.081g	0.41g	1.4mg	0.65g	1.9g	0g	0.16mg	10mg	0.081mg	0mcg	0mcg

1. Unsweetened

VEGETABLES

FOOD	SERVING SIZE	CALORIES	FAT	PROTEIN	SODIUM	FIBER	CARBO-HYDRATES	SUGAR	ZINC	CALCIUM	IRON	VITAMIN D	VITAMIN B_{12}
Alfalfa sprouts	1 cup	10	0g	1g	2mg	1g	1g	0g	0mg	11mg	0mg	0mcg	0mcg
Artichokes	1 medium	60	0g	4g	114mg	6.9g	13g	0g	0.63mg	56mg	1.6mg	0mcg	0mcg
Asparagus	1 cup	27	0.15g	2.7g	2.7mg	2.7g	5.3g	2.7g	1.3mg	32mg	2.7mg	0mcg	0mcg
Asparagus, steamed	½ cup	19.8	0.2g	2.2g	12.6mg	1.8g	3.7g	1.2g	0.5mg	20.7mg	0.8mg	0mcg	0mcg
Beans, baked	½ cup	120	0.5g	6g	480mg	6g	24g	9g	2.1mg	40mg	2.7mg	0mcg	0mcg
Beans, black	1 cup	227	0.9g	15.2g	1.7mg	15g	40.8g	0g	1.9mg	46.4mg	3.6mg	0mcg	0mcg
Beans, butter	½ cup canned	110	0.5g	6g	420mg	5g	19g	0g	0mg	60mg	1.79mg	0mcg	0mcg
Beans, cannellini	½ cup canned	154	0.44g	9.2g	6.6mg	6.6g	29g	0g	1.3mg	96mg	3.9mg	0mcg	0mcg
Beans, fava	1 cup canned	182	0.57g	13g	375mg	10g	31g	0g	2.6mg	67mg	2.6mg	0mcg	0mcg
Beans, garbanzo	¾ cup canned	213	2g	9g	534mg	7.1g	41g	0g	1.8mg	57mg	1.8mg	0mcg	0mcg
Beans, kidney	1 cup canned	210	2.6g	13g	759mg[2]	10g	38g	5.1g	0mg	87mg	2.6mg	0mcg	0mcg
Beans, lima	¼ cup uncooked	151	0.45	9.4g	8mg	8.5g	28g	4g	1.3mg	36mg	3.6mg	0mcg	0mcg
Beans, mung	¼ cup uncooked	180	0.6g	12g	7.8mg	8.4g	32g	3.4g	1.4mg	68mg	3.5mg	0mcg	0mcg
Beans, navy	½ cup canned	148	0.56g	9.9g	586mg	6.7g	27g	0.37g	1mg	62mg	2.4mg	0mcg	0mcg
Beans, pinto	1 cup cooked	205	2g	12g	23mg	12g	36g	0g	2.4mg	102mg	2.4mg	0mcg	0mcg
Beans, refried	1 cup	217	2.8g	12.9g	1,069mg	12.1g	36.3g	1.1g	1.5mg	78.6mg	4mg	0mcg	0mcg
Beans, yellow wax	1 cup	27	0.14g	1.6g	2.7mg	1.8g	6.1g	1.3g	0.39mg	35mg	1.2mg	0mcg	0mcg
Bean sprouts	1 cup	31	0g	3g	0mg	2g	6g	4g	0mg	0mg	0mg	0mcg	0mcg
Beets	1 cup	58	0.3g	2.7g	105mg	4.1g	14g	9.5g	0mg	22mg	1.4mg	0mcg	0mcg
Beetgreens	1 cup	8	0g	0.77g	87mg	1.5g	1.5g	0.38g	0mg	45mg	1.2mg	0mcg	0mcg
Bok choy	1 cup	20	0g	2g	90mg	2g	4g	0g	4.3mg	32mg	1.1mg	0mcg	0mcg
Broccoli, raw	1 cup	30.9	0.3g	2.6g	30mg	2.4g	6g	1.5g	0.4mg	42.8mg	0.7mg	0mcg	0mcg
Broccoli, steamed	1 stalk[1]	49	0.6g	3.3g	57.4mg	4.6g	10.1g	1.9g	0.6mg	56mg	0.9mg	0mcg	0mcg
Broccoli rabe	1 cup, chopped	8.8	0.2g	1.3g	13.2mg	1.1g	1.2g	0.2g	0.3mg	43.2mg	0.9mg	0mcg	0mcg
Brussels sprouts	1 cup	61	1g	4g	33mg	4g	14g	0g	0mg	56mg	2mg	0mcg	0mcg
Cabbage	1 cup	22	0.1g	0.91g	16mg	1.8g	5.5g	3.6g	0mg	43mg	0.91mg	0mcg	0mcg
Cauliflower	1 cup	25	0.1g	2g	30mg	2.5g	5.3g	2.4g	0.3mg	22mg	0.4mg	0mcg	0mcg
Carrots	1 cup	52.5	0.3g	1.2g	88.3mg	3.6g	12.3g	6.1g	0.3mg	42.2mg	0.4mg	0mcg	0mcg
Carrots, baby	3 oz	29.8	0.1g	0.5g	66.3mg	2.5g	7g	4g	0.1mg	27.2mg	0.8mg	0mcg	0mcg
Cauliflower	1 cup	25	0.11g	2g	30mg	3g	5g	2g	0mg	22mg	0mg	0mcg	0mcg
Celery	1 cup	14	0.22g	1g	81mg	2g	3g	2g	0mg	40mg	0mg	0mcg	0mcg
Chilies, Anaheim		18	0g	1.0g	3.0mg	1.0g	4.0g	2.0g	0mg	10mg	0.5mg	0mcg	0mcg
Chilies, poblano	1	13	0.1g	0.1g	1.9mg	1.1g	3.0g	1.5g	0.0mg	6.4mg	0.2mg	0mcg	0mcg
Chilies, red	1	18	0.2g	0.8g	4.0mg	0.7g	4.0g	2.4g	0.1mg	6.3mg	0.5g	0mcg	0mcg
Collardgreens	1 cup	11	0.16g	0.71g	7.1mg	1.4g	2.1g	0g	0mg	52mg	0mg	0mcg	0mcg
Corn on the cob	1 ear	155	3.4g	4.5g	29.2mg	0g	31.9g	0g	0.9mg	4.4mg	0.9mg	0mcg	0mcg
Cucumber	1 cucumber	45.1	0.3g	2g	6mg	1.5g	10.9g	5g	0.6mg	48.2mg	0.8mg	0mcg	0mcg
Edamame	1 cup	189	8.1g	16.9g	9,3mg	8.1g	15.8g	3.4g	2.1mg	97.6mg	3.5mg	0mcg	0mcg
Eggplant	1 cup	32.7	0.2g	0.8g	237mg	2.5g	8.1g	3.2g	0.1mg	5.9mg	0.2mg	0mcg	0mcg
Endives	2 cups	17	0.22g	1g	22mg	3g	3g	0g	1mg	52mg	1mg	0mcg	0mcg
Garlic	1 clove	4.5	0g	0.2g	0.5mg	0.1g	1g	0g	0mg	5.4mg	0.1mg	0mcg	0mcg

1. About 1 cup, 2. Rinse canned beans to minimize sodium

FOOD	SERVING SIZE	CALORIES	FAT	PROTEIN	SODIUM	FIBER	CARBO-HYDRATES	SUGAR	ZINC	CALCIUM	IRON	VITAMIN D	VITAMIN B_{12}
Kale	1 cup	33	0.67g	2g	29mg	1.3g	6.7g	0g	0mg	90mg	1.3mg	0mcg	0mcg
Kohlrabi	1 cup	36	0.15g	2.7g	27mg	5.4g	8.1g	4.1g	0mg	32mg	0mg	0mcg	0mcg
Leeks	1 cup	55	0.3g	1.8g	18mg	1.8g	13g	3.6g	0mg	54mg	1.8mg	0mcg	0mcg
Lentils	¼ cup[2]	170	0.53g	13g	2.9mg	15g	29g	0.96g	2.4mg	27mg	3.8mg	0mcg	0mcg
Lettuce, iceberg	1 cup	10.1	0.1g	0.6g	7.2mg	0.9g	2.3g	1.4g	0.1mg	13mg	0.3mg	0mcg	0mcg
Lettuce, romaine	1 cup	8	0.1g	0.6g	3.8mg	1g	1.5g	0.6g	0.1mg	15.5mg	0.5mg	0mcg	0mcg
Mushrooms, portabella	1 medium	29	0.25g	3.4g	6.8mg	2.3g	5.7g	2.3g	1.1mg	9.1mg	1.1mg	0mcg	0mcg
Mushrooms, shiitake	1 cup	81	0.32g	2.9g	5.8mg	2.9g	20g	5.8g	1.4mg	4.3mg	0mg	0mcg	0mcg
Mushroom, white button	1 cup	16	0.24g	2.1g	3.6mg	0.71g	2.1g	1.4g	0.71mg	2.1mg	0.71mg	0mcg	0mcg
Olives, green	1 oz	40.6	4.3g	0.3g	436mg	0.9g	1.1g	0.2g	0mg	14.6mg	0.1mg	0mcg	0mcg
Olives, kalamata	5 olives	20	2g	0g	330mg	0g	1g	0g	0mg	0mg	0mg	0mcg	0mcg
Okra	1 cup	31	0.11g	2g	8mg	3g	7g	1g	1mg	81mg	1mg	0mcg	0mcg
Onion, boiled pearl	1 cup	43	0g	0g	0mg	0g	1g	0g	0mg	3.1mg	0mg	0mcg	0mcg
Onion, red	1 onion	42	0g	0g	0mg	0g	1g	0g	0mg	3mg	1.2mg	0mcg	0mcg
Parsnips	1 cup	100	0.44g	1.3g	13mg	6.7g	24g	6.7g	1.3mg	48mg	1.3mg	0mcg	0mcg
Peas	1 cup	117	0.64g	7.2g	7.2mg	7.2g	20g	8.7g	1.4mg	36mg	1.4mg	0mcg	0mcg
Peas, black-eyed	1 cup canned	199	3.8g	6.6g	839mg	7.9g	40g	0g	2.5mg	41mg	3.4mg	0mcg	0mcg
Pepper, chili	1 pepper	18	0.2g	0.91g	4.1mg	0.91g	4.1g	2.3g	0mg	6.4mg	0.45mg	0mcg	0mcg
Pepper, jalapeño	1 pepper	4	0.14g	0.14g	0.14mg	0.42g	0.85g	0.42g	0mg	1.4mg	0.14mg	0mcg	0mcg
Pepper, green bell	1 cup	29.8	0.3g	1.3g	4.5mg	2.5g	6.9g	3.6g	0.2mg	14.9mg	0.5mg	0mcg	0mcg
Pepper, roasted red bell	1 oz	9.3	0g	0g	112mg	0.9g	3.7g	0.9g	0mg	0mg	1mg	0mcg	0mcg
Pepper, yellow bell	1 pepper	32	0g	1g	2mg	2g	8g	0g	0mg	11mg	1mg	0mcg	0mcg
Potatoes, Russet	1 small[3]	128	0.2g	3.5g	13.8mg	3g	29.2g	1.6g	0.5mg	20.7mg	1.5mg	0mcg	0mcg
Pumpkin	1 cup	30	0.13g	1.2g	1.2mg	1.2g	8.1g	1.2g	0mg	24mg	1.2mg	0mcg	0mcg
Rutabaga	1 cup	51	0.31g	1.4g	28mg	4.2g	11g	8.5g	0mg	66mg	1.4mg	0mcg	0mcg
Sweet potato	1 small[4]	54	0.1g	1.2g	21.6mg	2g	12.4g	3.9g	0.2mg	22.8mg	0.4mg	0mcg	0mcg
Spinach	1 cup	6.9	0.1g	0.9g	23.7mg	0.7g	1.1g	0.1g	0.2mg	29.7mg	0.8mg	0mcg	0mcg
Spinach, steamed	1 cup	41.4	0.5g	5.3g	126mg	4.3g	6.7g	0.8g	1.4mg	245mg	6.4mg	0mcg	0mcg
Squash, acorn	1 cup	56	0.16g	1.4g	4.2mg	2.8g	14g	0g	0mg	46mg	1.4mg	0mcg	0mcg
Squash[1]	1 cup	82	0.2g	1.8g	8.2mg	0g	21.5g	4g	0.3mg	84mg	1.2mg	0mcg	0mcg
Squash, summer	1 cup	18	0.25g	1.1g	2.3mg	1.1g	3.4g	2.3g	0mg	17mg	0mg	0mcg	0mcg
Squash, spaghetti	1 cup	41.9	0.4g	1g	27.9mg	2.2g	10g	3.9g	0.3mg	32.6mg	0.5mg	0mcg	0mcg
Swiss chard	1 cup	7	0g	0.71g	76mg	0.71g	1.4g	0.36g	0mg	18mg	0.71mg	0mcg	0mcg
Tomato	1 medium	22.1	0.2g	1.1g	6.2mg	1.5g	4.8g	3.2g	0.2mg	12.3mg	0.3mg	0mcg	0mcg
Turnips	1 large	51	0.2g	1.8g	122mg	3.6g	11g	7.3g	0mg	55mg	0mg	0mcg	0mcg
Water chestnuts	¼ cup	30	0g	0.31g	4.3mg	0.93g	7.4g	1.5g	0.31mg	3.4mg	0mg	0mcg	0mcg
Watercress	¼ cup	1	0g	0.17g	3.5mg	0g	0.086g	0g	0mg	10mg	0mg	0mcg	0mcg
Yams	1 cup	176	0.33g	3g	13mg	6g	42g	1.5g	0mg	25mg	1.5mg	0mcg	0mcg
Zucchini	1 cup	19.8	0.2g	1.5g	12.4mg	1.4g	4.2g	2.1g	0.4mg	18.6mg	0.4mg	0mcg	0mcg
Zucchini, sautéed	1 cup	28.8	0.1g	1.2g	5.4mg	2.5g	7.1g	3g	0.3mg	23.4mg	0.6mg	0mcg	0mcg

1. Oven-roasted butternut, 2. Uncooked, 3. 138grams, 4. 60grams

	YOUR FAVORITE FOODS												
FOOD	SERVING SIZE	CALORIES	FAT	PROTEIN	SODIUM	FIBER	CARBO-HYDRATES	SUGAR	ZINC	CALCIUM	IRON	VITAMIN D	VITAMIN B_{12}

YOUR FAVORITE FOODS													
FOOD	SERVING SIZE	CALORIES	FAT	PROTEIN	SODIUM	FIBER	CARBO-HYDRATES	SUGAR	ZINC	CALCIUM	IRON	VITAMIN D	VITAMIN B_{12}

FOOD	SERVING SIZE	CALORIES	FAT	PROTEIN	SODIUM	FIBER	CARBO-HYDRATES	SUGAR	ZINC	CALCIUM	IRON	VITAMIN D	VITAMIN B$_{12}$

YOUR FAVORITE FOODS

THE PLANNER

WEEK 1

Welcome to your new adventurous life as a vegan! You've stocked your pantry, cleared out any non-vegan foods from your refrigerator, and made a date with your kitchen. Week 1 should be the easiest week, as you'll be feeling motivated and excited. We'll keep it simple this week and ease you into it with lots of familiar foods, as well as plenty of hearty and satisfying meals to keep you feeling full.

Don't worry too much about portion size or nutrition just yet. If you're hungry, just eat! Now is the time to focus on you and your new lifestyle. Say no to any extra personal or professional commitments that may distract you, because you need to be focused on yourself and your new diet this week. Make sure you have plenty of time in the morning to eat breakfast and pack a lunch, and save a bit of extra time in the evening to relax and enjoy the process of cooking dinner.

If your friends and family are supportive, now's the time to let everyone know what you're doing. Knowing they're watching will help keep you honest. On the other hand, if you're surrounded by naysayers, don't feel like you have to talk about it.

Your goal this week? Take good care of yourself, but most importantly, enjoy eating all of the delicious, healthy foods!

MENU

BREAKFAST	LUNCH	SNACK	DINNER
2 slices whole grain bread, 1 T. peanut butter, 1 T. sugar-free jam, 1 banana	Veggie burger with ¼ tomato, ½ avocado sliced, 1 small bunch of kale on 2 slices of whole grain bread; 1 c. baked beans; 1 c. orange juice	Mixed vegetables (½ cucumber, 2 oz. baby carrots, ½ c. broccoli) with 3 T. hummus	1 c. **Basic Vegetable Marinara** with 1 c. whole grain pasta; side green salad with 2 c. romaine lettuce or kale, 1 tomato, and 1 diced cucumber, 2 T. **Goddess Dressing**

BASIC VEGETABLE MARINARA

Serves 6

This staple will come in handy to eat with pasta, as a dipping sauce, or in a casserole.

4 cloves garlic, minced	1 t. fresh parsley
1 carrot, sliced thin	2 T. chopped fresh basil
2 stalks celery, chopped	2 bay leaves
2 T. olive oil	½ c. canned corn
1 (28-oz.) can diced tomatoes	½ c. sliced black olives
1 (6-oz.) can tomato paste	1 T. balsamic vinegar
1 t. dried oregano	½ t. crushed red pepper flakes
	½ t. salt

1. Heat garlic, carrot, and celery in olive oil over medium heat, stirring frequently, for 4–5 minutes.
2. Reduce heat to medium low, then add tomatoes, tomato paste, oregano, parsley, basil, and bay leaves, stirring well to combine.
3. Cover and heat for at least 30 minutes, stirring frequently.
4. Add corn, olives, vinegar, red pepper flakes, and salt, and simmer for another 5 minutes, uncovered.
5. Remove bay leaves before serving.

PER SERVING Calories **143** Fat **7G** Protein **4G** Sodium **583MG** Fiber **4G** Carbohydrates **20G** Sugar **11G** Zinc **1MG** Calcium **70MG** Iron **3MG** Vit. D **0MCG** Vit. B$_{12}$ **0MCG**

IN A PINCH

Don't have time to make marinara from scratch? Take five minutes to heat a store-bought jar on the stove and add in frozen vegetables, Italian seasonings, and a bit of wine or balsamic vinegar for a fresh taste.

GODDESS DRESSING

Yields 1½ cups

Turn this zesty salad dressing into a dip for vegetables or a sandwich spread by reducing the amount of liquids.

⅔ c. tahini	1 clove garlic
¼ c. apple cider vinegar	¾ t. sugar
⅓ c. soy sauce	⅓ c. olive oil
2 t. lemon juice	

1. Process all the ingredients except olive oil together in a blender or food processor until blended.
2. With the blender or food processor on high speed, slowly add in the olive oil, blending for another full minute, allowing the oil to emulsify.
3. Chill in the refrigerator for at least 10 minutes before serving; dressing will thicken as it chills.

PER SERVING (2 T) Calories **131** Fat **12G** Protein **3G** Sodium **222MG** Fiber **1G** Carbohydrates **4G** Sugar **0G** Zinc **1MG** Calcium **25MG** Iron **1MG** Vit. D **0MCG** Vit. B$_{12}$ **0MCG**

What I Ate

DATE _____ | _____ | _____

TIME	FOOD ITEM	AMOUNT	CALORIES	FAT	CARBS	FIBER	PROTEIN
		TOTAL					

Today's Vegan Plate

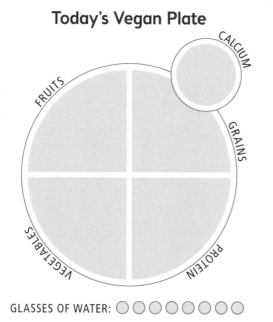

GLASSES OF WATER: ◯◯◯◯◯◯◯◯

Thoughts about Today

MENU

BREAKFAST	LUNCH	SNACK	DINNER
¾ c. whole grain cereal, 1 c. plant-based milk of your choice	Hummus (2 T.) sandwich with ½ cucumber, ½ c. sprouts, and 1 oz. roasted red peppers on 2 slices of whole grain bread	200 calories of whole grain chips with ½ c. salsa	1 c. Sun-Dried Tomato Risotto with Spinach, 1 c. Caramelized Baby Carrots

SUN-DRIED TOMATO RISOTTO WITH SPINACH

Serves 4

The tomatoes carry the flavor in this easy risotto—no butter, cheese, or wine are needed. But if you're a gourmand who keeps truffle, hazelnut, pine nut, or another gourmet oil on hand, now's the time to use it instead of the margarine.

1 yellow onion, diced	1 c. fresh chopped spinach
4 cloves garlic, minced	1 T. chopped fresh basil
2 T. olive oil	2 T. nutritional yeast
1½ c. Arborio rice	1 t. salt
6 c. vegetable broth, divided	1 t. black pepper
⅔ c. rehydrated sun-dried tomatoes, sliced	

1. Heat onion and garlic in olive oil until just soft, about 2–3 minutes. Add rice, and toast for 1 minute, stirring constantly.
2. Add ¾ cup vegetable broth and stir to combine. When most of the liquid has been absorbed, add another ½ cup, stirring constantly. Continue adding liquid ½ cup at a time (reserving ½ cup) until rice is cooked, about 20 minutes.
3. Add remaining broth, tomatoes, spinach, and basil, and reduce heat to low. Stir to combine well. Heat for 3–4 minutes until tomatoes are soft and spinach is wilted.
4. Stir in nutritional yeast. Taste, then season with salt and pepper. Risotto will thicken a bit as it cools.

PER SERVING Calories 326 Fat 8G Protein 9G Sodium 1,908MG Fiber 4G Carbohydrates 55G Sugar 6G Zinc 1MG Calcium 46MG Iron 4MG Vit. D 0MCG Vit. B$_{12}$ 2MCG

CARAMELIZED BABY CARROTS

Serves 4

Baby carrots have a natural sweetness when cooked, and this recipe turns them into a treat everyone will love!

4 c. baby carrots	2 T. vegan margarine
Water for boiling	2 T. brown sugar
1 t. lemon juice	¼ t. sea salt

1. Simmer carrots in water until just soft, about 8–10 minutes; do not overcook. Drain and drizzle with lemon juice.
2. Heat together carrots, margarine, brown sugar, and sea salt, stirring frequently until glaze forms and carrots are well coated, about 5 minutes.

PER SERVING Calories 130 Fat 6G Protein 1G Sodium 327MG Fiber 4G Carbohydrates 20G Sugar 14G Zinc 0MG Calcium 55MG Iron 1MG Vit. D 0MCG Vit. B$_{12}$ 0MCG

SUN-DRIED TOMATOES

If you're using dehydrated tomatoes, rehydrate them first by covering in water for at least 10 minutes, and add the soaking water to the broth. If you're using tomatoes packed in oil, add 2 T. of the oil to risotto at the end of cooking instead of the vegan margarine.

What I Ate

DATE [   ] | [   ] | [   ]

TIME	FOOD ITEM	AMOUNT	CALORIES	FAT	CARBS	FIBER	PROTEIN
	TOTAL						

Today's Vegan Plate

FRUITS / CALCIUM / GRAINS / PROTEIN / VEGETABLES

GLASSES OF WATER: ○○○○○○○○

Thoughts about Today

MENU

BREAKFAST	LUNCH	SNACK	DINNER
½ c. old fashioned oats with 1 c. blueberries, ¼ c. chopped almonds, and 2 t. maple syrup; 1 c. chocolate soy milk	2 pieces **Easy Vegan Pizza Bagels**, 1 c. sliced strawberries, 1 c. orange juice	1 (6") pita with 2 T. hummus	1½ c. **Black Bean and Butternut Squash Chili**

EASY VEGAN PIZZA BAGELS

Serves 4

Need a quick lunch or after-school snack for the kids? Pizza bagels to the rescue! For a real treat, grab some vegan pepperoni slices, such as Smart Deli Pepperoni from Lightlife or sausage crumbles from Gardein, to top them off. Add additional vegan toppings as desired.

⅓ c. tomato sauce
½ t. garlic powder
¼ t. salt
½ t. dried basil
½ t. dried oregano

4 whole grain (3") bagels, sliced in half
8 slices vegan cheese
¼ c. sliced mushrooms
¼ c. sliced black olives

1. Preheat oven to 325°F.
2. Combine tomato sauce, garlic powder, salt, basil, and oregano.
3. Spread sauce over each bagel half, and top with cheese, mushrooms, and olives.
4. Heat in oven for 8–10 minutes.

PER SERVING Calories **435** Fat **17G** Protein **14G** Sodium **1,168MG** Fiber **7G** Carbohydrates **60G** Sugar **8G** Zinc **1MG** Calcium **29MG** Iron **3MG** Vit. D **0MCG** Vit. B$_{12}$ **0MCG**

DON'T GO WITHOUT YOUR JOE!

You don't have to give up your daily cup-o'-joe when you go vegan! Try a soy- or coconut-milk creamer to whiten your brew, or use plain or vanilla soy milk with a bit of sugar. Chain coffeehouses such as Starbucks, Pret a Manger, and Peet's Coffee all offer milk alternatives. Similarly, it's unusual for local coffeehouses *not* to have plant-based milk options. If they don't, though, politely request that they start supplying them!

BLACK BEAN AND BUTTERNUT SQUASH CHILI

Serves 6

Squash is an excellent addition to a meat-free chili in this Southwestern-style dish.

1 onion, chopped
3 cloves garlic, minced
2 T. sunflower oil
1 medium butternut squash, peeled and chopped into chunks
2 (15-oz.) cans black beans, drained

1 (28-oz.) can stewed tomatoes, undrained
¾ c. water
1 T. chili powder
1 t. cumin
¼ t. cayenne pepper
½ t. salt
2 T. chopped fresh cilantro

1. In a large stockpot, sauté onion and garlic in oil until soft, about 4 minutes.
2. Reduce heat and add remaining ingredients, except cilantro.
3. Cover and simmer for 25 minutes. Uncover and simmer another 5 minutes. Top with fresh cilantro just before serving.

PER SERVING Calories **259** Fat **6G** Protein **11G** Sodium **532MG** Fiber **12G** Carbohydrates **46G** Sugar **9G** Zinc **1MG** Calcium **143MG** Iron **5MG** Vit. D **0MCG** Vit. B$_{12}$ **0MCG**

What I Ate

DATE [____] | [____] | [____]

TIME	FOOD ITEM	AMOUNT	CALORIES	FAT	CARBS	FIBER	PROTEIN
TOTAL							

Today's Vegan Plate

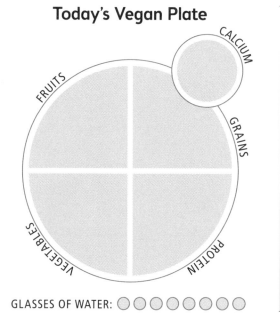

CALCIUM

FRUITS

GRAINS

VEGETABLES

PROTEIN

GLASSES OF WATER: ○○○○○○○○

Thoughts about Today

BREAKFAST	LUNCH	SNACK	DINNER
12 oz. **Chocolate Peanut Butter Banana Smoothie**	1½ c. leftover **Black Bean and Butternut Squash Chili** (see recipe in Week 1, Wed.); side green salad with 2 c. romaine lettuce or kale, 1 tomato, and 1 diced cucumber, 2 T. **Goddess Dressing** (see recipe in Week 1, Mon.); 1 c. orange juice	1 c. unsweetened applesauce, 1 oz. raisins	⅓ **Green Olive and Artichoke Focaccia Pizza**, 1 c. steamed cauliflower

CHOCOLATE PEANUT BUTTER BANANA SMOOTHIE

Serves 2

Yummy enough for a dessert, but healthy enough for breakfast, this smoothie is also a great protein boost after a workout. Replace the soy milk with another dairy-free milk if you prefer.

- 7–8 ice cubes
- 2 medium bananas
- 2 T. natural peanut butter
- 2 T. unsweetened cocoa powder
- 1 c. calcium-fortified unsweetened soy milk

Blend together all ingredients until smooth.

PER SERVING Calories **252** Fat **11G** Protein **10G** Sodium **48MG** Fiber **7G** Carbohydrates **36G** Sugar **16G** Zinc **1MG** Calcium **169MG** Iron **2MG** Vit. D **0MCG** Vit. B$_{12}$ **1MCG**

WHAT'S MISSING?

Feeling hungry or like you're just "missing something"? It may be water that you're craving. Keep a reusable water bottle by your side wherever you go—in the car, in the office, in the living room—to help make sure you're getting enough. Get in the habit of guzzling a big glass of water first thing in the morning to start your day well hydrated.

GREEN OLIVE AND ARTICHOKE FOCACCIA PIZZA

Serves 3

This gourmet vegan pizza has plenty of Italian seasonings. It's so flavorful, you won't miss the cheese at all. Add in mock meat toppings if you like!

- 1 vegan focaccia bread (12" diameter), sliced
- 1 T. olive oil
- ½ t. salt
- ½ t. dried rosemary
- ½ t. dried basil
- ⅓ c. tomato paste
- ½ c. chop sliced green olives
- ¾ c. chopped artichoke hearts
- ½ c. sliced button mushrooms
- 3 cloves garlic, minced
- ½ t. dried parsley
- ¼ t. dried oregano
- ½ t. red pepper flakes

1. Preheat oven to 400°F.
2. Drizzle focaccia with olive oil and sprinkle with salt, rosemary, and basil.
3. Spread a thin layer of tomato paste on the focaccia, then top with olives, artichoke hearts, mushrooms, and garlic.
4. Sprinkle with parsley, oregano, and red pepper flakes, then bake for 20 minutes, or until done.

PER SERVING Calories **361** Fat **16G** Protein **12G** Sodium **1,409MG** Fiber **4G** Carbohydrates **45G** Sugar **6G** Zinc **2MG** Calcium **82MG** Iron **6MG** Vit. D **0MCG** Vit. B$_{12}$ **0MCG**

What I Ate

DATE [   ] | [   ] | [   ]

TIME	FOOD ITEM	AMOUNT	CALORIES	FAT	CARBS	FIBER	PROTEIN
	TOTAL						

Today's Vegan Plate

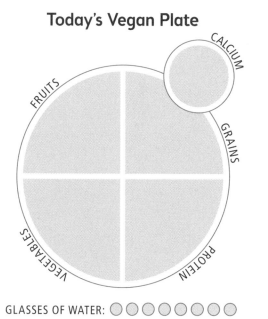

CALCIUM

FRUITS

GRAINS

VEGETABLES

PROTEIN

GLASSES OF WATER: ○○○○○○○○

Thoughts about Today

MENU

BREAKFAST	LUNCH	SNACK	DINNER
⅓ c. granola, 1 c. plant-based milk of your choice	⅓ leftover Green Olive and Artichoke Focaccia Pizza (see recipe in Week 1, Thurs.); side green salad with 2 c. romaine lettuce or kale, 1 tomato, and 1 diced cucumber, 2 T. Goddess Dressing (see recipe in Week 1, Mon.); 1 c. orange juice	Mixed fruit salad with ½ apple, ½ banana, ½ c. strawberries, and ½ c. pineapple; 1 oz. cashews	1¾ c. Italian White Bean and Fresh Herb Salad, 1 c. steamed spinach

ITALIAN WHITE BEAN AND FRESH HERB SALAD

Serves 4

Don't let the simplicity of this bean salad fool you. The fresh herbs marinate the beans to flavorful perfection. Feel free to substitute great northern beans for the cannellini beans.

2 (15-oz.) cans cannellini beans, drained and rinsed	3 large tomatoes, chopped
2 stalks celery, diced	½ c. sliced black olives
¼ c. chopped fresh parsley	2 T. lemon juice
¼ c. chopped fresh basil	1 t. salt
3 T. olive oil	1 t. black pepper
	¼ t. crushed red pepper flakes

1. In a large skillet, combine beans, celery, parsley, and basil with olive oil. Heat, stirring frequently, over low heat for 3 minutes until herbs are softened, but not cooked.
2. Remove from heat and stir in remaining ingredients, gently tossing to combine. Chill for at least 1 hour before serving.

PER SERVING Calories 302 Fat 14G Protein 12G Sodium 999MG Fiber 10G Carbohydrates 35G Sugar 4G Zinc 1MG Calcium 109MG Iron 3MG Vit. D 0MCG Vit. B₁₂ 0MCG

FRESH IS ALWAYS BEST

Cans are convenient, but dried beans are cheaper, need less packaging, add a fresher flavor, and, if you plan in advance, aren't much work at all to prepare. Place your beans in a large pot, and cover with plenty of water (more than you think you'll need), then allow them to sit for at least 2 hours. Overnight is fine. Drain the soaking water and simmer in fresh water for about an hour, then you're good to go! One cup of dried beans yields about 3 cups cooked. If you are often short on time, you may want to consider investing in an Instant Pot®, which can cook beans in under 30 minutes!

What I Ate

DATE [   ] | [   ] | [   ]

TIME	FOOD ITEM	AMOUNT	CALORIES	FAT	CARBS	FIBER	PROTEIN
TOTAL							

Today's Vegan Plate

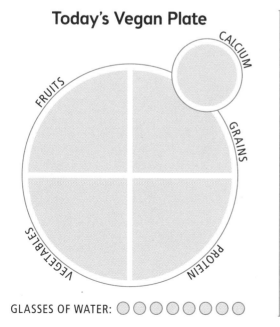

CALCIUM

FRUITS

GRAINS

VEGETABLES

PROTEIN

GLASSES OF WATER: ○○○○○○○○

Thoughts about Today

MENU

BREAKFAST	LUNCH	SNACK	DINNER
1 **Potato Poblano Breakfast Burrito**, 1 c. orange juice	Hummus wrap with ¼ c. tomatoes, ½ c. spinach, ½ c. sprouts, and 1 oz. olives in a large flour tortilla; 1 c. soy milk	1 c. edamame	1 c. **Asian Sesame Tahini Noodles**; 1 c. grilled pineapple; side green salad with 2 c. romaine lettuce or a leafy green of your preference, 1 tomato, 1 diced cucumber, 2 T. **Goddess Dressing** (see recipe in Week 1, Mon.)

POTATO POBLANO BREAKFAST BURRITOS

Serves 3

Wrap these filling burritos in foil for a great on-the-go breakfast. If the hot sauce is too spicy for your taste, use ketchup instead.

2 T. olive oil
2 small Yukon potatoes, diced small
2 poblano chilies, seeded and diced
1 t. chili powder
1 t. salt
1 t. black pepper
1 medium tomato, diced

⅔ c. vegan ground beef or sausage alternative, such as from Gardein, Lightlife or Beyond Meat
3 large flour tortillas, warmed
1 c. grated vegan cheese (Violife cheese is perfect for grating)
1 T. hot sauce

1. Heat olive oil in a pan and add potatoes and chilies, sautéing until potatoes are almost soft, about 6–7 minutes.
2. Add chili powder, salt and pepper, tomato, and meat alternative, and stir well to combine.
3. Continue cooking until potatoes and tomatoes are soft and meat alternative is cooked, another 4–5 minutes.
4. Wrap in warmed flour tortillas with vegan cheese and hot sauce.

PER SERVING Calories **659** Fat **33G** Protein **15G** Sodium **2,309MG** Fiber **6G** Carbohydrates **77G** Sugar **6G** Zinc **1MG** Calcium **198MG** Iron **5MG** Vit. D **0MCG** Vit. B$_{12}$ **0MCG**

ASIAN SESAME TAHINI NOODLES

Serves 4

A creamy and nutty Chinese-inspired noodle dish. If you don't have Asian-style noodles, such as lo mein or mei fun, on hand, spaghetti will do. You could also try zucchini noodles!

1 lb. Asian noodles
½ c. tahini
⅓ c. water
2 T. soy sauce
1 clove garlic, minced
2 t. fresh ginger, peeled and minced

2 T. rice vinegar
2 t. sesame oil
1 red bell pepper, sliced thin
3 scallions, chopped
¾ c. snow peas, chopped
¼ t. crushed red pepper flakes

1. Cook noodles according to package instructions, drain well.
2. Whisk or blend together tahini, water, soy sauce, garlic, ginger, and vinegar.
3. In a large skillet, heat oil, bell pepper, scallions, and snow peas for 2–3 minutes. Add tahini sauce and noodles, stirring well to combine.
4. Cook over low heat just until heated, about 2–3 minutes. Garnish with crushed red pepper flakes.

PER SERVING Calories **764** Fat **36G** Protein **16G** Sodium **1,786MG** Fiber **7G** Carbohydrates **94G** Sugar **9G** Zinc **3MG** Calcium **92MG** Iron **8MG** Vit. D **0MCG** Vit. B$_{12}$ **0MCG**

What I Ate

DATE [   ] | [   ] | [   ]

TIME	FOOD ITEM	AMOUNT	CALORIES	FAT	CARBS	FIBER	PROTEIN
		TOTAL					

Today's Vegan Plate

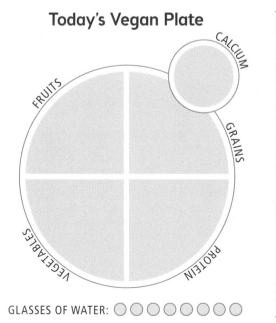

GLASSES OF WATER: ○○○○○○○○

Thoughts about Today

BREAKFAST	LUNCH	SNACK	DINNER
3 slices **Easy Vegan French Toast**, 1 c. strawberries, 1 c. soy milk	Banana and peanut butter sandwich on 2 slices toasted whole grain bread, 1 c. pineapple, 1 apple or 1 pear	1 c. soy yogurt with ⅓ c. granola, 1 c. orange juice	1½ c. **Bell Peppers Stuffed with Couscous**, ½ c. black beans, 1 c. steamed broccoli

EASY VEGAN FRENCH TOAST

Serves 4

Instead of drowning your French toast in powdered sugar and maple syrup, use a healthier sugar-free jam or some agave nectar for a satisfyingly sweet topping.

2 medium bananas
½ c. unsweetended soy
  milk
1 T. orange juice
1 T. maple syrup
¾ t. vanilla
1 T. all-purpose flour

1 t. cinnamon
½ t. nutmeg
1½ T. vegan margarine,
  such as Earth Balance,
  for frying
12 thick slices brioche
  bread

1. Using a blender or mixer, mix together bananas, soy milk, orange juice, maple syrup, and vanilla until smooth and creamy.
2. Whisk in flour, cinnamon, and nutmeg, and pour into a pie plate or shallow pan.
3. Heat vegan margarine in a large skillet.
4. Dip or spoon mixture over bread on both sides, and fry in hot oil until lightly golden brown on both sides, about 2–3 minutes.

PER SERVING Calories **529** Fat **31G** Protein **10G** Sodium **481MG** Fiber **4G** Carbohydrates **54G** Sugar **14G** Zinc **1MG** Calcium **95MG** Iron **3MG** Vit. D **1MCG** Vit. B$_{12}$ **1MCG**

BELL PEPPERS STUFFED WITH COUSCOUS

Serves 4

Baked stuffed peppers are always a hit with those who appreciate presentation, and this recipe takes very little effort.

4 c. water
3 c. couscous
2 T. olive oil
2 T. lemon juice
1 c. frozen peas, thawed

2 scallions, sliced
½ t. cumin
½ t. chili powder
4 green bell peppers

1. Preheat oven to 350°F.
2. Bring water to a boil and add couscous. Cover, turn off heat, and let sit for 10–15 minutes until couscous is cooked. Fluff with a fork.
3. Combine couscous with olive oil, lemon juice, peas, scallions, cumin, and chili powder.
4. Cut the tops off bell peppers and remove seeds, saving the tops.
5. Stuff couscous into bell peppers and place the tops back on, using a toothpick to secure, if needed.
6. Transfer to a baking dish and bake for 15 minutes.

PER SERVING Calories **618** Fat **8G** Protein **20G** Sodium **54MG** Fiber **11G** Carbohydrates **114G** Sugar **7G** Zinc **2MG** Calcium **60MG** Iron **3MG** Vit. D **0MCG** Vit. B$_{12}$ **0MCG**

What I Ate

DATE [ ] | [ ] | [ ]

TIME	FOOD ITEM	AMOUNT	CALORIES	FAT	CARBS	FIBER	PROTEIN
	TOTAL						

Today's Vegan Plate

CALCIUM

FRUITS

GRAINS

VEGETABLES

PROTEIN

GLASSES OF WATER: ○○○○○○○○

Thoughts about Today

JOURNAL

I FEEL:

MY GREATEST FOOD DISCOVERY THIS WEEK WAS:

THIS WEEK'S BIGGEST VEGAN CHALLENGE WAS:

NEW FOOD I'D LIKE TO TRY:

WHEN I LOOK BACK AT THIS WEEK, I MOST WANT TO REMEMBER:

HOW ARE YOU PROGRESSING TOWARD YOUR GOALS?

WEEK 2

You made it through Week 1! How are you feeling? You should feel proud of yourself. You've probably noticed a boost in energy thanks to eating a variety of nutrient-rich foods. Most people find that during the first couple of weeks of eating vegan they feel "lighter" or less sluggish mentally and physically. Food is moving through your digestive system more quickly, your body is happy with the abundance of nourishment it's receiving, and all those extra nutrients are flooding your system with energy. Is your skin a little brighter? Nails a little stronger? Are your pants a little looser? And don't forget about all the animals' lives you have saved in just a week. The environment thanks you!

Now that you know you can do it, Week 2 is going to be even easier. This week, we'll try out some foods that might be new to you, such as tofu and dairy substitutes, and you may start to notice some changes in your body. If you're used to eating a diet heavy in meats, dairy, and processed foods, your body will continue to adjust to this new easily digestible and nutritious diet—not to mention all the extra fiber you're getting! This may lead to feelings of bloating, or even feeling grumpy. Think of these as sort of food-withdrawal symptoms, because that's exactly what they are. The solution? Drink lots of water, grab a healthy snack, and let the feelings pass. Have a favorite movie handy to distract you, or catch up with a friend over tea.

Now is the time when you're more than likely feeling absolutely fantastic! Ready for Week 2? Let's do it!

MENU

BREAKFAST	LUNCH	SNACK	DINNER
1 (3") bagel with 2 T. hummus, 1 banana, 1 c. tomato juice (no salt added)	1¾ c. **Greek Salad with Vegan Feta Cheese**	1 apple, 1 oz. almonds	1 oz. **Sun-Dried Tomato Pesto** with 1 c. whole grain pasta, 1 c. steamed spinach with 16g nutritional yeast

GREEK SALAD WITH VEGAN FETA CHEESE

Serves 3

This colorful salad is a great go-to for lunch on a busy day.

¼ c. olive oil
2 T. balsamic vinegar
1 t. chopped fresh basil
½ t. dried oregano
½ t. salt
½ t. black pepper
1 8 oz. package of vegan feta cheese, such as from Violife

2 medium tomatoes, sliced
1 medium yellow bell pepper, chopped
1 large cucumber, sliced
½ red onion, diced
¼ c. kalamata olives, pitted

1. Whisk together olive oil, vinegar, basil, oregano, salt, and black pepper. Add crumbled feta, covering well with dressing. Allow to marinate for at least 1 hour.
2. Add remaining ingredients and gently toss to combine well.

PER SERVING Calories **488** Fat **43G** Protein **2G** Sodium **1,081MG** Fiber **3G** Carbohydrates **21G** Sugar **8G** Zinc **0G** Calcium **38MG** Iron **1MG** Vit. D **0MCG** Vit. B$_{12}$ **2MCG**

SUN-DRIED TOMATO PESTO

Yields 1 cup

You'll reach for this versatile spread again and again! If you don't have pine nuts, use walnuts.

⅓ c. sun-dried tomatoes
2 c. fresh basil leaves
½ c. pine nuts
3 cloves garlic

¼ c. nutritional yeast
½ t. salt
¼ t. black pepper
¼ c. olive oil

1. If using dehydrated sun-dried tomatoes, reconstitute in water until soft and pliable, about 15 minutes.
2. Purée together all ingredients, adding oil last to achieve desired consistency.

PER SERVING (¼ CUP) Calories **255** Fat **24G** Protein **5G** Sodium **290MG** Fiber **2G** Carbohydrates **7G** Sugar **2G** Zinc **2MG** Calcium **49MG** Iron **2MG** Vit. D **0MCG** Vit. B$_{12}$ **4MCG**

What I Ate

DATE [   ] | [   ] | [   ]

TIME	FOOD ITEM	AMOUNT	CALORIES	FAT	CARBS	FIBER	PROTEIN
		TOTAL					

Today's Vegan Plate

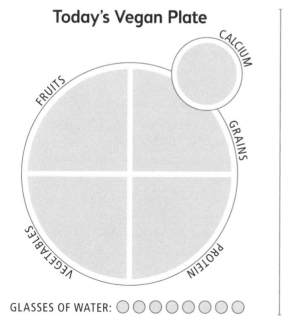

FRUITS

CALCIUM

GRAINS

VEGETABLES

PROTEIN

Thoughts about Today

GLASSES OF WATER: ○○○○○○○○○

BREAKFAST	LUNCH	SNACK	DINNER
2 c. **Strawberry Protein Smoothie**, 1 c. chocolate soy milk	Vegan sandwich with 1 oz. **Sun-Dried Tomato Pesto** (see recipe in Week 2, Mon.), 1 oz. avocado, 1 tomato slice, and ½ c. sprouts on 2 slices of whole grain bread; 1 c. tomato juice (no salt added); 3 oz. baby carrots with 1 T. hummus	200 calories of whole grain chips with ¼ c. **Black Bean Guacamole**	1½ c. **Curried Rice and Lentils**

STRAWBERRY PROTEIN SMOOTHIE

Serves 2

This sweet and simple smoothie is a protein-packed way to start your day. You can use another nondairy milk if you prefer.

½ c. frozen strawberries
1 scoop plant-based protein powder, such as Vega or Orgain
8 oz. lite, unsweetened coconut milk
1 medium banana
¾ c. orange juice
3–4 ice cubes
1 T. agave nectar

Blend together all ingredients until smooth and creamy.

PER SERVING Calories **198** Fat **4G** Protein **7G** Sodium **54MG** Fiber **4G** Carbohydrates **38G** Sugar **25G** Zinc **0MG** Calcium **66MG** Iron **2MG** Vit. D **1MCG** Vit. B$_{12}$ **1MCG**

BLACK BEAN GUACAMOLE

Yields 2 cups

The addition of black beans to this guacamole boosts the fiber and protein content.

1 (15-oz.) can black beans, drained and rinsed
3 avocados
1 T. lime juice
3 scallions, chopped
1 large tomato, diced
2 cloves garlic, minced
½ t. chili powder
¼ t. salt
1 T. chopped fresh cilantro

1. Using a fork or a potato masher, mash beans in a medium-sized bowl just until they are halfway mashed, leaving some texture.
2. Combine all remaining ingredients, and mash together until mixed.
3. Allow to sit for at least 10 minutes before serving to allow the flavors to set.
4. Gently mix again just before serving.

PER SERVING (2 T.) Calories **35** Fat **2G** Protein **1G** Sodium **35MG** Fiber **2G** Carbohydrates **3G** Sugar **0G** Zinc **0MG** Calcium **9MG** Iron **0MG** Vit. D **0MCG** Vit. B$_{12}$ **0MCG**

CURRIED RICE AND LENTILS

Serves 4

Use fresh green peas if possible when you make this—they bring a bright and refreshing flavor.

1½ c. brown rice
1 c. dried lentils
1 medium tomato, diced
1 c. green peas
3½ c. water
1 T. curry powder
½ t. cumin
½ t. turmeric
½ t. garlic powder
1 t. salt
1 t. black pepper

1. Combine all ingredients except salt and pepper in a large soup or stockpot. Bring to a slow simmer, then cover and cook for 20 minutes, stirring occasionally until rice is done and liquid is absorbed.
2. Add salt and pepper.

PER SERVING Calories **477** Fat **3G** Protein **20G** Sodium **614MG** Fiber **12G** Carbohydrates **94G** Sugar **3G** Zinc **3MG** Calcium **65MG** Iron **6MG** Vit. D **0MCG** Vit. B$_{12}$ **0MCG**

What I Ate

DATE [   ] | [   ] | [   ]

TIME	FOOD ITEM	AMOUNT	CALORIES	FAT	CARBS	FIBER	PROTEIN
		TOTAL					

Today's Vegan Plate

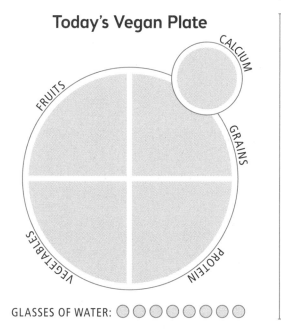

GLASSES OF WATER: ○○○○○○○○○

Thoughts about Today

BREAKFAST	LUNCH	SNACK	DINNER
¾ c. whole grain cereal, 1 c. plant-based milk, 1 c. sliced fresh pineapple	1½ c. leftover **Curried Rice and Lentils** (see recipe in Week 2, Tues.) with 1 medium tomato added	½ (3") bagel with 1 T. hummus	½ block **Easy Barbecue Baked Tofu**; 1 medium steamed sweet potato; side green salad with 2 c. romaine lettuce, 1 tomato, and 1 diced cucumber, 2 T. **Goddess Dressing** (see recipe in Week 1, Mon.)

EASY BARBECUE BAKED TOFU

Serves 2

The spice mixture in this recipe gives the tofu loads of flavor. Serve topped with extra sauce, if preferred.

1½ t. paprika	¼ t. smoked paprika
1 t. cumin	¼ t. black pepper
1 t. chili powder	1 14 oz. container extra-firm tofu, well pressed
1 t. garlic powder	1½ T. olive oil
½ t. kosher salt	¾ c. barbecue sauce

1. Preheat oven to 350°F. Mix spices in separate bowl. Slice tofu into squares or strips about ¾" thick. Coat tofu in olive oil and spice mixture.
2. Brush a layer of barbecue sauce on a baking sheet. Arrange tofu slices in a single layer, and brush well with a layer of barbecue sauce.
3. Bake for 30–40 minutes or until tofu is lightly crisped and sauce is baked on.

PER SERVING Calories **419** Fat **15G** Protein **22G** Sodium **1,680MG** Fiber **5G** Carbohydrates **50G** Sugar **35G** Zinc **0MG** Calcium **205MG** Iron **5MG** Vit. D **0MCG** Vit. B$_{12}$ **0MCG**

SHAKEN, NOT STIRRED

Before you pour that glass of nondairy milk, shake it up! The calcium in these drinks tends to settle at the bottom of the carton, so to get the best bone-boosting effect, shake before you drink. If you're a heavy smoker or coffee drinker, consider taking a supplement, as these inhibit absorption of several nutrients.

What I Ate

DATE [   ] | [   ] | [   ]

TIME	FOOD ITEM	AMOUNT	CALORIES	FAT	CARBS	FIBER	PROTEIN
	TOTAL						

Today's Vegan Plate

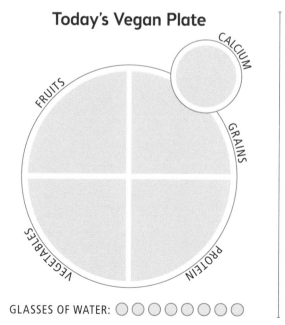

GLASSES OF WATER: ○○○○○○○○

Thoughts about Today

MENU

BREAKFAST	LUNCH	SNACK	DINNER
1 large flour tortilla wrap with 1 T. nondairy cream cheese and 1 c. sliced strawberries, 1 c. chocolate soy milk	Barbecue tofu sandwiches from leftover **Easy Barbecue Baked Tofu** (see recipe in Week 2, Wed.) with 1 T. vegan mayonnaise, ¼ tomato (sliced), and ¼ c. iceberg lettuce on 2 slices of whole grain bread; 1 apple or 1 pear; 1 c. plant-based milk of your choice	1 c. popcorn with 16g nutritional yeast	2 **Portabella and Pepper Fajitas** topped with ½ c. vegetable salsa and 2 T. vegan sour cream, 1 c. steamed broccoli

PORTABELLA AND PEPPER FAJITAS

Serves 2

Top these fajitas with vegan sour cream (try Follow Your Heart sour cream or Tofutti sour cream), salsa, avocado, or other vegan choice.

2 T. olive oil
2 large portabella mush-rooms, cut into strips
1 medium green bell pep-per, cut into strips
1 medium red bell pep-per, cut into strips
1 medium onion, cut into strips

¾ t. chili powder
¼ t. cumin
⅛ t. hot sauce
1 T. chopped fresh cilantro
4 large flour tortillas, warmed

1. Heat olive oil in a large skillet and add mush-rooms, bell peppers, and onion. Allow to cook for 3–5 minutes until vegetables are almost done.
2. Add chili powder, cumin, and hot sauce, and stir to combine. Cook for 2–3 more minutes until mushrooms and peppers are soft. Remove from heat and stir in fresh cilantro.
3. Layer the mushrooms and peppers in flour tortillas.

PER SERVING Calories **660** Fat **26G** Protein **17G** Sodium **1,114MG** Fiber **11G** Carbohydrates **91G** Sugar **17G** Zinc **2MG** Calcium **242MG** Iron **7MG** Vit. D **1MCG** Vit. B$_{12}$ **0MCG**

COOKING FOR OMNIVORES?

If your family and friends still insist on eating a bit of meat, offer to cook their favorite meal in a vegan way. With the abundance of plant-based foods, it's never been easier (or tastier) to veganize meals. Show your family and friends by example just how great a vegan diet is!

What I Ate

DATE [   ] | [   ] | [   ]

TIME	FOOD ITEM	AMOUNT	CALORIES	FAT	CARBS	FIBER	PROTEIN
TOTAL							

Today's Vegan Plate

CALCIUM

FRUITS

GRAINS

VEGETABLES

PROTEIN

Thoughts about Today

GLASSES OF WATER: ○ ○ ○ ○ ○ ○ ○ ○

MENU

BREAKFAST	LUNCH	SNACK	DINNER
1½ c. **Tropical Breakfast Couscous**, 1 banana	1⅛ c. **Spicy Southwestern Two-Bean Salad**, 1 apple or 1 sliced mango, 1 c. orange juice	1 slice whole grain toast with ½ T. peanut butter	1 c. **Artichoke and Olive Puttanesca**, 1 c. steamed spinach

TROPICAL BREAKFAST COUSCOUS

Serves 2

You won't question couscous for breakfast after you try this sweet fruit-filled dish. Garnish with fresh fruit for great nutrition, flavor, and presentation! If you don't have pineapple juice, just use orange juice.

1 c. lite coconut milk, unsweetened

1 c. pineapple juice

1 c. couscous

½ t. vanilla

2 T. maple syrup

1. In a small saucepan, heat coconut milk and juice until just about to simmer. Do not boil.
2. Add couscous and heat for 1 minute. Stir in vanilla, cover, and turn off heat. Allow to sit, covered, for 5 minutes until couscous is cooked.
3. Fluff couscous with a fork and stir in maple syrup.

PER SERVING Calories **472** Fat **3** Protein **12G** Sodium **21MG** Fiber **5G** Carbohydrates **97G** Sugar **25G** Zinc **1MG** Calcium **108MG** Iron **2MG** Vit. D **2MCG** Vit. B$_{12}$ **2MCG**

SPICY SOUTHWESTERN TWO-BEAN SALAD

Serves 6

The heat in this dish is offset by the bell peppers and lime juice, so add more cayenne pepper and chili powder if you like!

1 (15-oz.) can black beans, drained and rinsed

1 (15-oz.) can kidney beans, drained and rinsed

1 medium red bell pepper, chopped

1 large tomato, diced

⅔ c. corn (fresh, canned, or frozen)

1 medium red onion, diced

⅓ c. olive oil

¼ c. lime juice

½ t. chili powder

½ t. garlic powder

¼ t. cayenne pepper

½ t. salt

¼ c. chopped fresh cilantro

1. In a large bowl, combine black beans, kidney beans, bell pepper, tomato, corn, and onion.
2. In a separate small bowl, whisk together olive oil, lime juice, chili powder, garlic powder, cayenne pepper, and salt.
3. Pour oil mixture over bean mixture, tossing to coat. Stir in fresh cilantro.
4. Chill for at least 1 hour before serving to allow flavors to mingle. Gently toss again just before serving.

PER SERVING Calories **251** Fat **13G** Protein **8G** Sodium **397MG** Fiber **4G** Carbohydrates **27G** Sugar **3G** Zinc **1MG** Calcium **67MG** Iron **2MG** Vit. D **0MCG** Vit. B$_{12}$ **0MCG**

ARTICHOKE AND OLIVE PUTTANESCA

Serves 4

For dinner tonight, head to Italy for a tasty meal of puttanesca. The aromatic dish will have you coming back for seconds!

3 cloves garlic, minced

2 T. olive oil

1 (14-oz.) can diced tomatoes, drained

¼ c. sliced black olives

¼ c. sliced green olives

1 c. chopped artichoke hearts

2 T. capers

½ t. red pepper flakes

½ t. dried basil

¾ t. dried parsley

¼ t. salt

1 (12-oz.) package of long pasta, such as spaghetti, prepared according to package instructions

2 T. grated Parmesan cheese (such as the Violife dairy free cheese)

1. Heat garlic in olive oil in a large, deep skillet for 2–3 minutes. Reduce heat and add remaining ingredients, except pasta and Parmesan.
2. Cook over low heat, uncovered, for 10 minutes until most of the liquid from tomatoes is absorbed.
3. Toss with pasta. Serve with Parmesan cheese.

PER SERVING Calories **485** Fat **12G** Protein **16G** Sodium **1,039MG** Fiber **6G** Carbohydrates **77G** Sugar **6G** Zinc **1MG** Calcium **86MG** Iron **5MG** Vit. D **0MCG** Vit. B$_{12}$ **0MCG**

What I Ate

DATE [   ] | [   ] | [   ]

TIME	FOOD ITEM	AMOUNT	CALORIES	FAT	CARBS	FIBER	PROTEIN
		TOTAL					

Today's Vegan Plate

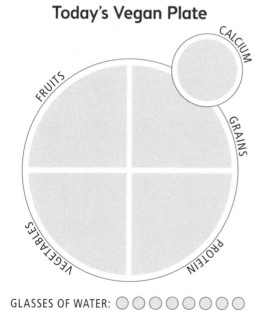

GLASSES OF WATER: ○ ○ ○ ○ ○ ○ ○ ○

Thoughts about Today

MENU

BREAKFAST	LUNCH	SNACK	DINNER
1 c. **Chili Masala Tofu Scramble**	1 c. leftover **Artichoke and Olive Puttanesca** (see recipe in Week 2, Fri.)	1 medium apple, sliced, with ½ T. peanut butter; ½ oz. raisins	7 oz. **Cuban Black Beans, Sweet Potatoes, and Rice**; 1 c. steamed broccoli

CHILI MASALA TOFU SCRAMBLE

Serves 2

Tofu scramble is a versatile vegan breakfast. This version adds chili and curry for extra flavor. Toss in vegetables you have on hand—tomatoes, spinach, kale, or diced broccoli work well.

- 1 (14-oz.) block extra-firm tofu, pressed
- 1 small onion, diced
- 2 cloves garlic, minced
- 2 T. olive oil
- 1 small red chili pepper, minced and seeded
- 1 medium green bell pepper, chopped
- ¾ c. sliced shiitake mushrooms
- 1 T. soy sauce
- 1 t. curry powder
- ½ t. cumin
- ¼ t. turmeric
- 1 t. nutritional yeast

1. Crumble tofu or cut into 1" cubes.
2. Sauté onion and garlic in olive oil for 1–2 minutes until onion is soft.
3. Add tofu, chili pepper, bell pepper, and mushrooms, stirring well to combine.
4. Add remaining ingredients, except nutritional yeast, and combine well. Allow to cook until tofu is lightly browned, about 6–8 minutes.
5. Remove from heat and stir in nutritional yeast.

PER SERVING Calories **372** Fat **24G** Protein **23G** Sodium **456MG** Fiber **5G** Carbohydrates **16G** Sugar **6G** Zinc **1MG** Calcium **177MG** Iron **4MG** Vit. D **0MCG** Vit. D$_{12}$ **1MCG**

WRAP IT UP

Leftover tofu scramble makes an excellent lunch, or you can wrap leftovers (or planned-overs!) in a warmed flour tortilla to make breakfast-style burritos with salsa or beans. Why isn't it called "scrambled tofu" instead of "tofu scramble" if it's an alternative for scrambled eggs? This is one of the great conundrums of veganism.

CUBAN BLACK BEANS, SWEET POTATOES, AND RICE

Serves 6

Stir some plain steamed rice right into the pot, or serve it on the side of these well-seasoned beans. This simple dish is packed full of protein, with tons of garlic and cumin flavors!

- 3 cloves garlic, minced
- 2 large sweet potatoes, peeled and chopped small
- 1 medium onion, diced
- 2 T. olive oil
- 2 (15-oz.) cans black beans, drained
- ¾ c. vegetable broth
- 1 T. chili powder
- 1 t. paprika
- 1 t. cumin
- 1 T. lime juice
- ½ T. hot sauce
- 2 c. cooked rice
- ¼ c. fresh cilantro

1. In a large skillet or soup pot, sauté garlic, sweet potatoes, and onion in olive oil for 2–3 minutes.
2. Reduce heat to medium low and add beans, vegetable broth, chili powder, paprika, and cumin. Bring to a simmer, cover, and allow to cook for 25–30 minutes until sweet potatoes are soft.
3. Stir in lime juice and hot sauce. Serve hot over rice topped with cilantro.

PER SERVING Calories **398** Fat **7G** Protein **16G** Sodium **613MG** Fiber **13G** Carbohydrates **70G** Sugar **4G** Zinc **2MG** Calcium **152MG** Iron **4MG** Vit. D **0MCG** Vit. B$_{12}$ **0MCG**

What I Ate

DATE ⬚ | ⬚ | ⬚

TIME	FOOD ITEM	AMOUNT	CALORIES	FAT	CARBS	FIBER	PROTEIN
		TOTAL					

Today's Vegan Plate

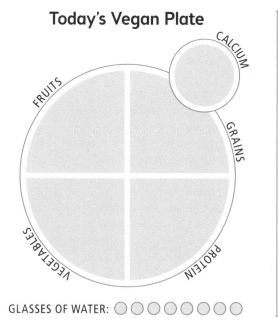

GLASSES OF WATER: ◯ ◯ ◯ ◯ ◯ ◯ ◯ ◯

Thoughts about Today

MENU

BREAKFAST	LUNCH	SNACK	DINNER
2 oz. store-bought polenta panfried in 1 t. olive oil with ½ c. salsa, 1 c. orange juice	7 oz. leftover Cuban Black Beans, Sweet Potatoes, and Rice (see recipe in Week 2, Sat.)	175 calories of whole grain chips with ¼ c. leftover Black Bean Guacamole (see recipe in Week 2, Tues.)	1½ c. Basic Tofu-Spinach Lasagna; side green salad with 2 c. romaine lettuce, 1 tomato, and 1 diced cucumber, 2 T. Goddess Dressing (see recipe in Week 1, Mon.)

BASIC TOFU-SPINACH LASAGNA

Serves 6

Seasoned tofu takes the place of ricotta cheese, and the spinach adds some tasty greens. Fresh parsley adds flavor, and with store-bought sauce, it's quick to get in the oven!

1 (14-oz.) block firm tofu
1 (14-oz.) block soft tofu
1 (12-oz.) block silken tofu
¼ c. nutritional yeast
1 T. lemon juice
1 T. soy sauce
1 t. garlic powder
2 t. dried basil
3 T. chopped fresh parsley

1 t. salt
2 (10-oz.) packages frozen chopped spinach, thawed
4 c. spaghetti sauce
1 (16-oz.) package lasagna noodles, cooked according to package instructions

1. In a large bowl, mash together firm tofu, soft tofu, silken tofu, nutritional yeast, lemon juice, soy sauce, garlic powder, basil, parsley, and salt until combined and crumbly like ricotta cheese. Stir in spinach.
2. Preheat oven to 350°F.
3. To assemble the lasagna, spread about ⅔ cup tomato sauce on the bottom of a lasagna pan, then add a layer of one third of the noodles.
4. Spread about half of the tofu mixture on top of the noodles, followed by another layer of sauce. Place a second layer of noodles on top, followed by the remaining tofu and more sauce. Finish it off with a third layer of noodles and the rest of the sauce.
5. Cover and bake for 25–30 minutes.

PER SERVING Calories 487 Fat 9G Protein 31G Sodium 1,627MG Fiber 10G Carbohydrates 72G Sugar 8G Zinc 2MG Calcium 373MG Iron 8MG Vit. D 0MCG Vit. B$_{12}$ 0MCG

READY-TO-GO POLENTA

Look for tubed polenta at the grocery store—it can usually be found in the refrigerated produce section (look near the tofu), or sometimes in the pasta aisle. Prepared polenta is already cooked, so all you need to do is fry it up in a sauté pan with some dairy-free butter.

What I Ate

DATE | | |

TIME	FOOD ITEM	AMOUNT	CALORIES	FAT	CARBS	FIBER	PROTEIN
		TOTAL					

Today's Vegan Plate

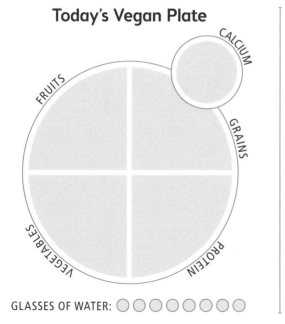

GLASSES OF WATER: ○ ○ ○ ○ ○ ○ ○ ○

Thoughts about Today

REVIEW

I FEEL:

MY GREATEST FOOD DISCOVERY THIS WEEK WAS:

THIS WEEK'S BIGGEST VEGAN CHALLENGE WAS:

NEW FOOD I'D LIKE TO TRY:

WHEN I LOOK BACK AT THIS WEEK, I MOST WANT TO REMEMBER:

HOW ARE YOU PROGRESSING TOWARD YOUR GOALS?

WEEK 3

By now, you've gotten used to cooking at home a bit more, and the excitement and newness of it all may have started to wear off as you begin settling into your new routine. Focus on small, positive changes to keep you motivated this week. Take a minute to browse through your notes from Week 1 and look at just how far you've come. How do you feel?

Eating vegan will begin to seem more normal to you now, and your friends and family will soon stop paying attention to your new habits. But don't let this new daily grind make you think the fun is over—you've still got lots of new food options to explore! You've tried tofu a few times, and you know what great variety the vegetable kingdom has to offer. Now you're ready to expand your options even further. This week, we'll continue experimenting with tofu, and try a few other new foods too. Are you ready to try some mock meats?

Give your taste buds a chance to adjust to the newness of meat substitutes. Some are startlingly similar in terms of flavor and texture. For instance, the Beyond Burger by plant-based company Beyond Meat boasts the ability to look, cook, and taste just like a beef burger. Not all mock meats are the same, so try a few different brands to find one that you like, or vary your preparation technique. For example, if you find you don't like microwaved vegan sausage patties, try pan frying them in a bit of oil. Veganism is all about trying new things!

MENU

BREAKFAST	LUNCH	SNACK	DINNER
1 English muffin with 1 vegan sausage patty, ¼ medium tomato, and 2 (1-oz.) avocado slices; 1 c. oat milk	1 baked potato with 2 T. vegan sour cream and ½ c. frozen mixed vegetables	2 oz. almonds, 1 oz. dried apricots, 1 c. orange juice	1½ c. **Potatoes "Au Gratin" Casserole**, 1 c. **Maple-Glazed Roast Veggies**

POTATOES "AU GRATIN" CASSEROLE

Serves 4

A classic dish—veganized! You won't have many leftovers after you taste this rich dish.

4 medium red potatoes	2 t. onion powder
1 medium onion, chopped	1 t. garlic powder
1 T. vegan margarine	2 T. nutritional yeast
2 T. all-purpose flour	1 t. lemon juice
2 c. unsweetened soy milk	½ t. salt
	¾ t. paprika
	½ t. black pepper

1. Preheat oven to 375°F.
2. Slice potatoes into thin coins and arrange half the slices in a casserole or baking dish. Layer half of the onion on top of the potatoes.
3. Melt margarine over low heat and add flour, stirring to make a paste. Add soy milk, onion powder, garlic powder, nutritional yeast, lemon juice, and salt, stirring to combine. Stir over low heat until sauce has thickened, about 2–3 minutes.
4. Pour half of sauce over potatoes and onions, then layer the remaining potatoes and onions on top of the sauce. Pour the remaining sauce on top.
5. Sprinkle with paprika and pepper.
6. Cover and bake for 45 minutes, and an additional 10 minutes, uncovered.

PER SERVING Calories **329** Fat **6G** Protein **19G** Sodium **440MG** Fiber **9G** Carbohydrates **51G** Sugar **5G** Zinc **4MG** Calcium **190MG** Iron **4MG** Vit. D **0MCG** Vit. B$_{12}$ **26MCG**

MAPLE-GLAZED ROAST VEGGIES

Serves 5

This delicious maple glaze can also be used as a salad dressing or a glaze for a mock meat. Get creative!

3 carrots, chopped	1 t. salt, divided
2 small parsnips, peeled and chopped	1 t. black pepper, divided
2 medium sweet potatoes, peeled and chopped	⅓ c. maple syrup
	2 T. Dijon mustard
2 T. olive oil	1 T. balsamic vinegar
	½ t. hot sauce

1. Preheat oven to 400°F.
2. On a large baking sheet, spread out chopped carrots, parsnips, and sweet potatoes. Drizzle with olive oil and season with ¼ teaspoon salt and ¼ teaspoon pepper. Roast for 40 minutes, tossing once, halfway through.
3. In a small bowl, whisk together maple syrup, Dijon mustard, balsamic vinegar, hot sauce, and remaining salt and pepper.
4. Transfer the roasted vegetables to a large bowl and toss well with the maple mixture.

PER SERVING Calories **191** Fat **6G** Protein **2G** Sodium **669MG** Fiber **4G** Carbohydrates **33G** Sugar **18G** Zinc **1MG** Calcium **61MG** Iron **1MG** Vit. D **0MCG** Vit. B$_{12}$ **0MCG**

What I Ate

DATE [   ] | [   ] | [   ]

TIME	FOOD ITEM	AMOUNT	CALORIES	FAT	CARBS	FIBER	PROTEIN
	TOTAL						

Today's Vegan Plate

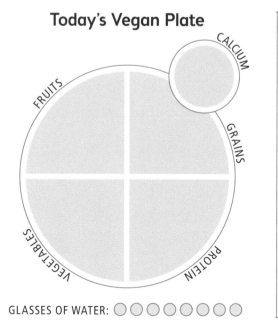

CALCIUM

FRUITS

GRAINS

VEGETABLES

PROTEIN

GLASSES OF WATER: ○○○○○○○○

Thoughts about Today

MENU

BREAKFAST	LUNCH	SNACK	DINNER
¾ c. whole grain cereal, 1 c. cashew milk, 1 banana or 1 c. blueberries	1 c. leftover **Maple-Glazed Roast Veggies** (see recipe in Week 3, Mon.), 1 c. store-bought tomato soup	1 oz. banana chips	1 **Tofu and Portabella Enchilada**; ½ c. black beans; side green salad with 2 c. romaine lettuce, 1 diced tomato, 1 diced cucumber, 2 T. **Goddess Dressing** (see recipe in Week 1, Mon.)

TOFU AND PORTABELLA ENCHILADAS

Serves 8

Turn up the heat by adding some fresh minced or canned chilies. If you love cheese, add a handful of grated vegan cheese to the filling as well as on top.

1 (14-oz.) block firm tofu, diced small
5 portabella mushrooms, chopped
1 medium onion, diced
3 cloves garlic, minced
2 T. vegetable oil
2 t. chili powder
½ c. sliced black olives
1 (15-oz.) can enchilada sauce
8 large flour tortillas

1. Preheat oven to 350°F.
2. In a large skillet, heat tofu, mushrooms, onion, and garlic in oil until tofu is just lightly sautéed, about 4–5 minutes. Add chili powder and heat for 1 more minute, stirring to coat well.
3. Remove from heat and add black olives and ⅓ cup enchilada sauce, and combine well.
4. Spread a thin layer of enchilada sauce in the bottom of a baking pan or casserole dish.
5. Place about ¼ cup of the tofu and mushrooms in each flour tortilla and roll, placing snugly in the baking dish. Top with remaining enchilada sauce, coating the tops of each tortilla well.
6. Bake for 25–30 minutes.

PER SERVING Calories **357** Fat **13G** Protein **14G** Sodium **1,085MG** Fiber **6G** Carbohydrates **48G** Sugar **10G** Zinc **1MG** Calcium **178MG** Iron **4MG** Vit. D **0MCG** Vit. B$_{12}$ **0MCG**

What I Ate

DATE [   ] | [   ] | [   ]

TIME	FOOD ITEM	AMOUNT	CALORIES	FAT	CARBS	FIBER	PROTEIN
		TOTAL					

Today's Vegan Plate

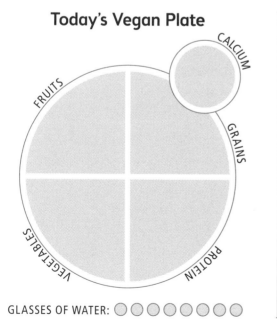

GLASSES OF WATER: ○○○○○○○○

Thoughts about Today

BREAKFAST	LUNCH	SNACK	DINNER
Peanut butter oatmeal (½ c. oatmeal with 1 T. peanut butter), 1 c. chocolate soy milk, 1 apple	1 leftover Tofu and Portabella Enchiladas (see recipe in Week 3, Tues.), 1 c. tomato juice (no salt added), 1 banana	3 oz. baby carrots dipped in 2 T. Goddess Dressing (see recipe in Week 1, Mon.), 1 c. strawberries	1 c. Indian Spiced Chickpeas with Spinach, 1 c. brown rice

INDIAN SPICED CHICKPEAS WITH SPINACH

Serves 3

This is a mild recipe, suitable for the whole family, but if you want to turn up the heat, toss in some fresh minced chilies or a hearty dash of cayenne pepper. It's enjoyable as is for a side dish, or piled on top of rice or another grain, such as quinoa or red rice, for a main meal.

1 medium onion, chopped	3 medium tomatoes, puréed, or ⅔ c. tomato paste
2 cloves garlic, minced	
2 T. vegan margarine	½ t. curry
¾ t. coriander	¼ t. turmeric
1 t. cumin	¼ t. salt
1 (15-oz.) can chickpeas, undrained	1 T. lemon juice
	1 bunch fresh spinach

1. In a large skillet, sauté onions and garlic in margarine until almost soft, about 2 minutes.
2. Reduce heat to medium low and add coriander and cumin. Toast the spices, stirring, for 1 minute.
3. Add chickpeas with liquid, tomatoes, curry, turmeric, and salt, and bring to a slow simmer. Allow to cook until most of the liquid has been absorbed, about 10–12 minutes, stirring occasionally, then add lemon juice.
4. Add spinach and stir to combine. Cook just until spinach begins to wilt, about 1 minute. Serve immediately.

PER SERVING Calories **254** Fat **11G** Protein **10G** Sodium **565MG** Fiber **10G** Carbohydrates **33G** Sugar **9G** Zinc **1MG** Calcium **156MG** Iron **4MG** Vit. D **0MCG** Vit. B$_{12}$ **0MCG**

What I Ate

DATE [   ] | [   ] | [   ]

TIME	FOOD ITEM	AMOUNT	CALORIES	FAT	CARBS	FIBER	PROTEIN
		TOTAL					

Today's Vegan Plate

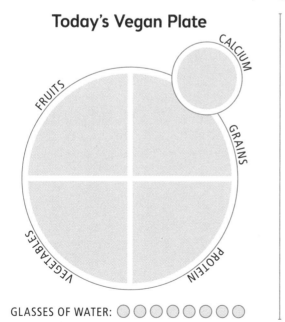

GLASSES OF WATER: ○○○○○○○○○

Thoughts about Today

MENU

BREAKFAST	LUNCH	SNACK	DINNER
1 c. Pumpkin Protein Smoothie, 1 c. canned pineapple, diced	2 Easy Vegan Pizza Bagels (see recipe in Week 1, Wed.) with 13 slices vegan pepperoni	2 oz. cashews, 1 c. orange juice	1 vegan chicken patty burger (try BOCA Original Chik'n Vegan Patties) with ¼ medium tomato, ¼ c. kale, and 1 T. vegan mayonnaise on 2 slices of whole wheat bread; 1 c. Vegan Ambrosia Fruit Salad; 1 ear corn; 1 c. almond milk

PUMPKIN PROTEIN SMOOTHIE

Serves 2

This smoothie brings together classic cool-weather favorites in one yummy drink. If you don't have pumpkin pie spice, use ⅛ teaspoon each of cinnamon, nutmeg, and allspice.

½ c. pumpkin purée
1 c. unsweetened soy milk
¼ c. plain soy yogurt

1 medium banana
5–6 ice cubes
¼ t. pumpkin pie spice
1 T. maple syrup

Blend all ingredients together until smooth and creamy.

PER SERVING Calories 316 Fat 6G Protein 11G Sodium 102MG Fiber 8G Carbohydrates 60G Sugar 35G Zinc 1MG Calcium 432MG Iron 4MG Vit. D 1MCG Vit. B$_{12}$ 3MCG

VEGAN PROTEIN SHAKES

By eating a balanced plant-based diet, you are already getting the nutrients you need. But if you work out, checking out vegan protein powders wouldn't be a bad idea. Health food stores as well as grocery stores sell a variety of vegan protein powders that you can add to a smoothie for all your muscle-building needs. Look for hemp protein powder or flax meal blends; just 3 teaspoons of hemp protein powder contains approximately 15 grams of protein!

VEGAN AMBROSIA FRUIT SALAD

Serves 5

You can use any type of yogurt, grapes, or nuts in this dish—tailor it to your taste buds.

1 (6-oz.) container vanilla vegan yogurt
1 (20-oz.) can pineapple tidbits, drained
1 medium apple, chopped small
1 c. grapes, any kind

1 (11-oz.) can mandarin oranges, drained
1 c. vegan mini marshmallows (try Dandies Mini Vanilla Marshmallows)
½ c. chopped walnuts
⅔ c. unsweetended flaked coconut

Gently toss all ingredients except nuts and coconut. Allow to chill for at least 1 hour. Top with flaked nuts and coconut before serving.

PER SERVING Calories 335 Fat 20G Protein 6G Sodium 28MG Fiber 5G Carbohydrates 40G Sugar 30G Zinc 1MG Calcium 88MG Iron 2MG Vit. D 0MCG Vit. B$_{12}$ 0MCG

What I Ate

DATE _____ | _____ | _____

TIME	FOOD ITEM	AMOUNT	CALORIES	FAT	CARBS	FIBER	PROTEIN
		TOTAL					

Today's Vegan Plate

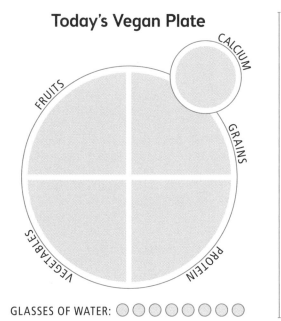

GLASSES OF WATER: ○○○○○○○○○

Thoughts about Today

MENU

BREAKFAST	LUNCH	SNACK	DINNER
1 c. leftover **Vegan Ambrosia Fruit Salad** (see recipe in Week 3, Thurs.), 1 c. soy hot chocolate	Sandwich with 2 slices vegan deli meats (try Tofurky or Lightlife deli slices); side green salad with 2 c. romaine lettuce, 1 tomato, 1 diced cucumber, and 2 T. **Goddess Dressing** (see recipe in Week 1, Mon.)	Mixed vegetables (½ cucumber, 2 oz. baby carrots, ½ c. broccoli) with 2 T. hummus	¾ c. **Baked Teriyaki Tofu Cubes** with 1 c. soba noodles

BAKED TERIYAKI TOFU CUBES

Serves 3

Cut tofu into wide slabs or triangular cutlets for a main dish, or smaller cubes to add to a salad, or just for an appetizer or snack. If you are short on time, consider buying premade vegan teriyaki sauce. If you've never cooked tofu before, this is a supereasy foolproof recipe to start with

⅓ c. soy sauce	2 T. riced wine vinegar
4 T. brown sugar	¼ c. maple syrup
⅔ c. water	¾ t. garlic powder
½ t. ground ginger	1 (14-oz.) block extra-
½ t. crushed red pepper	firm tofu, cut into ¼" cubes

1. Preheat oven to 375°F.
2. Mix all ingredients together, except for tofu, and let reduce by half. Remove from heat, then toss tofu in sauce. Coat well and bake for 10 minutes.

PER SERVING Calories **287** Fat **7G** Protein **16G** Sodium **1,577MG** Fiber **2G** Carbohydrates **41G** Sugar **35G** Zinc **1MG** Calcium **154MG** Iron **3MG** Vit. D **0MCG** Vit. B$_{12}$ **0MCG**

HOMEMADE BAKED TOFU

It's hard to go wrong with any flavor of homemade baked tofu. Use just about any store-bought salad dressing (be sure to check for any animal ingredients!), teriyaki sauce, barbecue sauce, or steak marinades. Thicker dressings may need to be thinned with a bit of water first, and to get the best glazing action, make sure there's a bit of sugar added. Another tip? Most baked tofu recipes will work just as well on an indoor electric grill in about a third of the time.

What I Ate

DATE ⬚ | ⬚ | ⬚

TIME	FOOD ITEM	AMOUNT	CALORIES	FAT	CARBS	FIBER	PROTEIN
	TOTAL						

Today's Vegan Plate

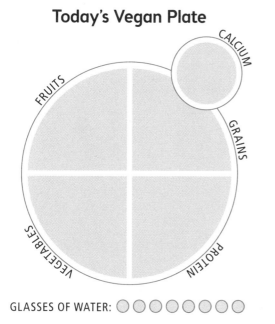

CALCIUM

FRUITS

GRAINS

VEGETABLES

PROTEIN

GLASSES OF WATER: ○○○○○○○○

Thoughts about Today

MENU

BREAKFAST	LUNCH	SNACK	DINNER
1½ c. **Chili Masala Tofu Scramble** (see recipe in Week 2, Sat.)	1½ c. **Sesame Snow Pea Rice Salad**	½ c. **Chili Cheese Dip** with about 200 calories of whole grain chips	Vegan burritos with ½ c. vegan ground beef substitute, ½ medium tomato, ¼ c. shredded lettuce

SESAME SNOW PEA RICE SALAD

Serves 4

The leftovers from this rice pilaf can be enjoyed chilled the next day as a cold rice salad.

4 c. cooked rice
2 T. olive oil
1 T. sesame oil
2 T. soy sauce
3 T. apple cider vinegar
1 t. sugar

1 c. snow peas, chopped
¾ c. baby corn, chopped
½ c. diced red peppers
3 scallions, chopped
2 T. chopped fresh parsley
½ t. sea salt

1. In a large pot over low heat, combine rice, olive oil, sesame oil, soy sauce, vinegar, and sugar, stirring well to combine.
2. Add snow peas, baby corn, red peppers, and scallions, and heat until warmed through and vegetables are lightly cooked, stirring frequently so the rice doesn't burn.
3. While still hot, stir in fresh parsley and season with sea salt.

PER SERVING Calories **389** Fat **11G** Protein **7G** Sodium **736MG** Fiber **3G** Carbohydrates **64G** Sugar **5G** Zinc **1MG** Calcium **38MG** Iron **4MG** Vit. D **0MCG** Vit. B$_{12}$ **0MCG**

EDA-WHAT?

You're probably familiar with the lightly steamed and salted edamame served as an appetizer at Japanese restaurants, but you may be surprised to learn that many grocers sell shelled edamame in the frozen foods section. Edamame, baby green soybeans, are a great source of unprocessed soy protein and make a great snack.

CHILI CHEESE DIP

Serves 5

This dip comes together quickly when you have unexpected guests. Dip with vegetable sticks or whole grain chips.

1 (15.5-oz.) can red kidney beans, drained
1 (1.25-oz.) packet chili seasoning
¼ c. nutritional yeast
1 (4-oz.) can yellow corn, drained

1 (8-oz.) container non-dairy cream cheese (try Tofutti or Follow Your Heart cream cheese alternatives)
½ c. seitan chorizo (try Upton's Naturals Chorizo Seitan)
¼ t. salt
1 T. sliced scallions for garnish

Mix together all ingredients until well combined. Heat in microwave for 1 minute, if desired, and serve.

PER SERVING Calories **289** Fat **15G** Protein **17G** Sodium **890MG** Fiber **7G** Carbohydrates **26G** Sugar **5G** Zinc **1MG** Calcium **61MG** Iron **2MG** Vit. D **0MCG** Vit. B$_{12}$ **4MCG**

What I Ate

DATE ___ | ___ | ___

TIME	FOOD ITEM	AMOUNT	CALORIES	FAT	CARBS	FIBER	PROTEIN
TOTAL							

Today's Vegan Plate

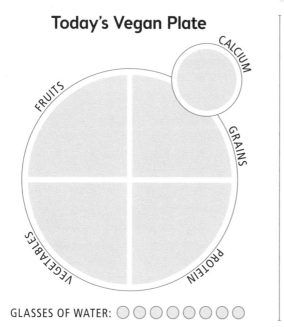

FRUITS
CALCIUM
GRAINS
VEGETABLES
PROTEIN

GLASSES OF WATER: ○○○○○○○○

Thoughts about Today

MENU

BREAKFAST	LUNCH	SNACK	DINNER
3 **Vegan Pancakes** with 1 c. fresh strawberries	1 c. **Edamame Salad**, 3 oz. baby carrots with 1 T. hummus	½ (3") bagel with 2 T. guacamole; ¼ medium tomato, sliced; 1 oz. pecans	1½ c. **Spanish Artichoke and Zucchini Paella**, 1 c. steamed spinach with 16g nutritional yeast

VEGAN PANCAKES

Yields I dozen pancakes

Add blueberries to this batter for a sweet treat!

1 c. all-purpose flour	½ **medium banana**
1 T. sugar	1 t. vanilla
1¾ t. baking powder	1 c. unsweetened soy
¼ t. salt	milk

1. Mix together flour, sugar, baking powder, and salt in a large bowl.
2. In a separate small bowl, mash banana with a fork. Add vanilla and whisk until smooth. Add soy milk and stir to combine.
3. Add soy milk mixture to the dry ingredients, stirring until combined.
4. Grease frying pan with oil or vegan butter and heat over medium heat. Drop batter about 3 T. at a time and heat until bubbles appear on surface, about 2–3 minutes. Flip and cook other side until lightly golden brown.

PER SERVING (1 PANCAKE) Calories **54** Fat **0G** Protein **2G** Sodium **109MG** Fiber **0G** Carbohydrates **11G** Sugar **2G** Zinc **0MG** Calcium **76MG** Iron **1MG** Vit. D **0MCG** Vit. B$_{12}$ **0MCG**

EDAMAME SALAD

Serves 4

Edamame beans are high in protein. Plus, they don't contain cholesterol and are low in calories.

2 c. frozen shelled edamame, thawed and drained	3 T. chopped fresh cilantro
	3 T. olive oil
1 medium red bell pepper, diced	2 T. red wine vinegar
	1 t. soy sauce
¾ c. frozen organic corn kernels	1 t. chili powder
	2 t. lemon juice

1. Combine edamame, bell pepper, corn, and cilantro in a large bowl.
2. Whisk together olive oil, vinegar, soy sauce, chili powder, and lemon juice. Combine with edamame and chill for at least 1 hour.

PER SERVING Calories **220** Fat **15G** Protein **11G** Sodium **100MG** Fiber **5G** Carbohydrates **15G** Sugar **4G** Zinc **1MG** Calcium **55MG** Iron **2MG** Vit. D **0MCG** Vit. B$_{12}$ **0MCG**

SPANISH ARTICHOKE AND ZUCCHINI PAELLA

Serves 4

Paella is a traditional Spanish rice dish, usually cooked with saffron. This tasty vegan version uses artichokes, zucchini, and turmeric instead.

3 cloves garlic, minced	½ c. artichoke hearts, chopped
1 medium yellow onion, diced	
	2 medium zucchinis, sliced
1 c. white rice	
1 (15-oz.) can diced tomatoes and drained	2 c. vegetable broth
	1 T. paprika
1 medium green bell pepper, chopped	½ t. turmeric
	¾ t. dried parsley
1 medium red bell pepper, chopped	½ t. salt

1. In a large skillet, heat garlic and onion in olive oil for 3–4 minutes. Add rice, stirring well to coat, and heat for 1 minute.
2. Add tomatoes, bell peppers, artichokes, and zucchini, stirring to combine. Add vegetable broth and remaining ingredients, cover, and simmer for 15–20 minutes, or until rice is done.

PER SERVING Calories **298** Fat **1G** Protein **9G** Sodium **891MG** Fiber **6G** Carbohydrates **64G** Sugar **12G** Zinc **2MG** Calcium **78MG** Iron **5MG** Vit. D **0MCG** Vit. B$_{12}$ **0MCG**

What I Ate

DATE [   ] | [   ] | [   ]

TIME	FOOD ITEM	AMOUNT	CALORIES	FAT	CARBS	FIBER	PROTEIN
		TOTAL					

Today's Vegan Plate

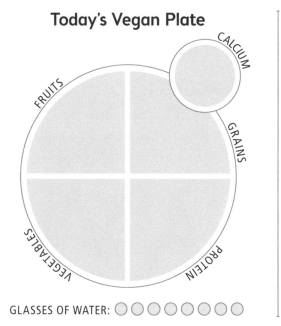

CALCIUM

FRUITS

GRAINS

VEGETABLES

PROTEIN

GLASSES OF WATER: ○○○○○○○○

Thoughts about Today

REVIEW

I FEEL:

MY GREATEST FOOD DISCOVERY THIS WEEK WAS:

THIS WEEK'S BIGGEST VEGAN CHALLENGE WAS:

NEW FOOD I'D LIKE TO TRY:

WHEN I LOOK BACK AT THIS WEEK, I MOST WANT TO REMEMBER:

HOW ARE YOU PROGRESSING TOWARD YOUR GOALS?

WEEK 4

By the end of this week, you'll have been vegan for nearly a whole month! This is a great milestone. Are you proud of yourself? You should be! By eating a vegan diet for just one month, you've saved 33,000 gallons of water, 900 square feet of forest, 1,200 pounds of grain, and 30 animals' lives. Behavioral studies suggest that it takes just over two months to establish new daily habits, so you are well on your way to fully making the change. This week, while things are settling into more of a routine, focus on how far you've come, and take a look back at what got you going in the first place. Your internal motivation and commitment to your goals will be your strength for the next couple of weeks.

Take time to review your original reasons for going vegan. Was it an online video about factory farming that inspired you to eat a more compassionate diet? Rewatch that video this week to keep yourself motivated. Was it an interview with a celebrity touting the miracle health and beauty benefits of a plant-based diet? Reread that interview. Tweet it, post it to *Facebook*, and keep it handy to keep you motivated, inspired, and educated. Revisit the goals that you wrote down before day one. Is it time to update them again?

After nearly a month, you're likely to have noticed a change in your tastes and preferences. This week, try out new whole grains as well as more vegan substitutes. Try different brands and flavors of vegan cheese to see which you like best, and watch out for hidden milk in the form of casein. Check out the bulk grain bins at your natural foods store to buy as little or as much as you need and for the best prices.

MENU

BREAKFAST	LUNCH	SNACK	DINNER
¾ c. whole grain cereal, 1 c. soy milk	½ c. **Eggless Egg Salad** on 2 slices whole grain bread with 1 slice tomato and ½ c. sprouts, mixed vegetables (½ cucumber, 2 oz. baby carrots, ½ c. broccoli) with 2 T. hummus	1 leftover **Vegan Pancake** (see recipe in Week 3, Sun.) with 1 T. peanut butter, 2 oz. banana chips	1½ c. **Pumpkin and Lentil Curry with Quinoa**

EGGLESS EGG SALAD

Serves 4

The relish, mustard, chives, and vegan bacon bits in this recipe pack a ton of flavor into the tofu.

- 1 (14-oz.) block firm tofu
- 1 (14-oz.) block silken tofu
- ½ c. vegan mayonnaise
- ⅓ c. sweet pickle relish
- ¾ t. apple cider vinegar
- ½ stalk celery, diced
- 2 T. minced onion
- 1½ T. Dijon mustard
- 2 T. chopped chives
- 2 T. vegan bacon bits
- 1 t. paprika

1. In a medium-sized bowl, use a fork to mash tofu together with the rest of the ingredients, except bacon bits and paprika.
2. Chill for at least 15 minutes before serving to allow flavors to mingle.
3. Garnish with vegan bacon bits and paprika just before serving.

PER SERVING Calories **172** Fat **8G** Protein **14G** Sodium **222MG** Fiber **2G** Carbohydrates **12G** Sugar **7G** Zinc **0MG** Calcium **204MG** Iron **2MG** Vit. D **0MCG** Vit. B$_{12}$ **0MCG**

PUMPKIN AND LENTIL CURRY WITH QUINOA

Serves 3

Adding pumpkin to this curry dish creates a mellow flavor and adds extra nutritional benefits.

- 1 medium yellow onion, chopped
- 2 c. puréed pumpkin
- 2 T. olive oil
- 1 T. curry powder
- 1 t. cumin
- ½ t. red pepper flakes
- 2 whole cloves
- 3 c. water
- 1 c. lentils
- 2 medium tomatoes, chopped
- 10 fresh green beans, trimmed and chopped
- ¾ c. unsweetened lite coconut milk
- 1½ c. cooked quinoa, prepared according to package

1. Sauté onion and pumpkin in olive oil until onion is soft, about 4 minutes. Add curry powder, cumin, red pepper, and cloves, and toast for 1 minute, stirring frequently.
2. Reduce heat slightly and add water and lentils. Cover and cook for about 10–12 minutes, stirring occasionally.
3. Uncover and add tomatoes, green beans, and coconut milk, stirring well to combine. Heat uncovered for 4–5 more minutes, just until tomatoes and beans are cooked.
4. Serve over cooked quinoa.

PER SERVING Calories **531** Fat **14G** Protein **24G** Sodium **32MG** Fiber **18G** Carbohydrates **84G** Sugar **12G** Zinc **4MG** Calcium **148MG** Iron **9MG** Vit. D **1MCG** Vit. B$_{12}$ **1MCG**

What I Ate

DATE ░░░░ | ░░░░ | ░░░░

TIME	FOOD ITEM	AMOUNT	CALORIES	FAT	CARBS	FIBER	PROTEIN
	TOTAL						

Today's Vegan Plate

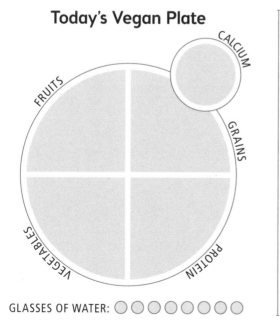

GLASSES OF WATER: ◯◯◯◯◯◯◯◯

Thoughts about Today

MENU

BREAKFAST	LUNCH	SNACK	DINNER
1 serving **Vanilla Date Breakfast Smoothie**	1½ c. leftover **Pumpkin and Lentil Curry with Quinoa** (see recipe in Week 4, Mon.), ½ c. frozen mixed vegetables with 2 T. salad dressing	1 oz. rice cakes with 1 T. almond butter	1 c. **Gingered Bok Choy and Tofu Stir-Fry**, 1 c. brown rice

VANILLA DATE BREAKFAST SMOOTHIE

Serves 1

Adding dates to a basic soy milk and fruit smoothie adds a blast of unexpected sweetness. Soaking your dates first will help them process a little quicker and results in a smoother consistency. Try putting a second banana in the freezer overnight and use that instead of the ice cubes. You can also throw in a scoop of your favorite protein powder.

4 dates
Water for soaking
¾ c. unsweetened soy milk

1 large frozen banana
6 ice cubes
1 t. vanilla extract

1. Cover dates with water and allow to soak for at least 10 minutes. This makes them softer and easier to blend.
2. Discard the soaking water and add dates and all other ingredients to the blender.
3. Process until smooth; about 1 minute on medium speed.

PER SERVING Calories **281** Fat **3G** Protein **7G** Sodium **66MG** Fiber **6G** Carbohydrates **58G** Sugar **39G** Zinc **1MG** Calcium **246MG** Iron **1MG** Vit. D **0MCG** Vit. B$_{12}$ **2MCG**

GINGERED BOK CHOY AND TOFU STIR-FRY

Serves 3

Dark leafy bok choy is a highly nutritious vegetable that can be found in well-stocked groceries, serving as an excellent source of iron, potassium, calcium, and magnesium. Keep an eye out for light green baby bok choy, which are a bit more tender but carry a similar flavor.

3 T. soy sauce
2 T. lime juice
1 T. fresh ginger, minced
1 (14-oz.) block extra-firm tofu, well pressed
2 T. olive oil

1 medium head bok choy or 4 small baby bok choys
½ t. sugar
½ t. sesame oil

1. Whisk together soy sauce, lime juice, and ginger in a shallow pan. Cut tofu into cubes, and marinate for at least 1 hour. Drain, reserving marinade.
2. In a large skillet or wok, sauté tofu in olive oil for 3–4 minutes.
3. Carefully add reserved marinade, bok choy, and sugar, stirring well to combine.
4. Cook, stirring, for 3–4 more minutes, or until bok choy is done. Drizzle with sesame oil and serve over rice.

PER SERVING Calories **270** Fat **17G** Protein **19G** Sodium **1,067MG** Fiber **5G** Carbohydrates **13G** Sugar **5G** Zinc **1MG** Calcium **407MG** Iron **5MG** Vit. D **0MCG** Vit. B$_{12}$ **0MCG**

What I Ate

DATE [   ] | [   ] | [   ]

TIME	FOOD ITEM	AMOUNT	CALORIES	FAT	CARBS	FIBER	PROTEIN
		TOTAL					

Today's Vegan Plate

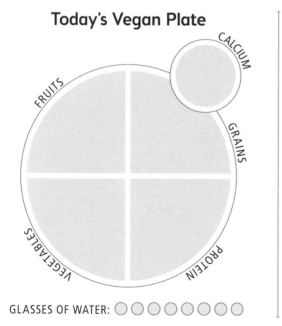

GLASSES OF WATER: ○○○○○○○○

Thoughts about Today

MENU

BREAKFAST	LUNCH	SNACK	DINNER
1 c. soy yogurt with ⅓ c. granola	½ c. leftover Gingered Bok Choy and Tofu Stir-Fry (see recipe in Week 4, Tues.), 1 c. brown rice	1 c. unsweetened applesauce, 1½ oz. mixed dried fruit (½ oz. raisins, ½ oz. dried cranberries, ½ oz. dried apricots)	1½ c. Bulgur Wheat Tabouli with 2 Easy Falafel Patties and 1 T. tahini

BULGUR WHEAT TABOULI

Serves 4

Though you'll need to adjust the cooking time, of course, you can try this tabouli recipe with just about any whole grain. Bulgur wheat is traditional, but quinoa, millet, or amaranth would also work.

1¼ c. boiling water	½ c. chopped fresh mint
1 c. bulgur wheat	½ c. chopped fresh
3 T. olive oil	parsley
¼ c. lemon juice	1 (15-oz.) can chickpeas,
1 t. garlic powder	drained
½ t. sea salt	2 large tomatoes, diced
½ t. black pepper	1 medium cucumber,
3 scallions, chopped	peeled and chopped

1. Pour boiling water over bulgur wheat. Cover, and allow to sit for 30 minutes, or until bulgur wheat is soft.
2. Toss bulgur wheat with olive oil, lemon juice, garlic powder, and salt, stirring well to coat. Combine with remaining ingredients, adding in tomatoes last.
3. Allow to chill for at least 1 hour before serving.

PER SERVING Calories 346 Fat 13G Protein 11G Sodium 477MG Fiber 11G Carbohydrates 52G Sugar 7G Zinc 2MG Calcium 99MG Iron 3MG Vit. D 0MCG Vit. B$_{12}$ 0MCG

EASY FALAFEL PATTIES

Serves 4

Falafel is a deep-fried ball, typically made from ground chickpeas, offering lots of protein and fiber. Health food stores sell a vegan instant falafel mix, but it's not very much work at all to make your own from scratch.

1 (15-oz.) can chickpeas, well drained	Egg substitute for 1 egg (try Bob's Red Mill
½ red onion, minced	Vegan Egg Replacer
1 T. all-purpose flour	or Follow Your Heart's
1 t. cumin	VeganEgg)
¾ t. garlic powder	¼ c. chopped fresh
¾ t. salt	parsley
	2 T. chopped fresh cilantro

1. Preheat oven to 375°F.
2. Place chickpeas in a large bowl and mash with a fork until coarsely mashed. Or pulse in a food processor until chopped.
3. Combine chickpeas with onion, flour, cumin, garlic, salt, and egg substitute, mashing together to combine. Add parsley and cilantro.
4. Shape mixture into 1"-thick patties (or 2" balls) and bake in oven for 15 minutes, or until crisp. Falafel can also be fried in oil for about 5–6 minutes on each side.

PER SERVING Calories 117 Fat 2G Protein 6G Sodium 609MG Fiber 5G Carbohydrates 19G Sugar 4G Zinc 1MG Calcium 52MG Iron 2MG Vit. D 0MCG Vit. B$_{12}$ 0MCG

What I Ate

DATE [   ] | [   ] | [   ]

TIME	FOOD ITEM	AMOUNT	CALORIES	FAT	CARBS	FIBER	PROTEIN
		TOTAL					

Today's Vegan Plate

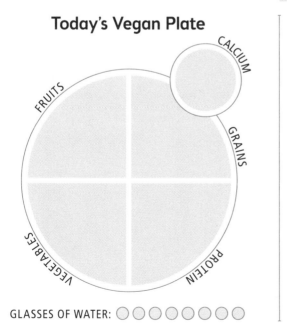

GLASSES OF WATER: ○○○○○○○○

Thoughts about Today

MENU

BREAKFAST	LUNCH	SNACK	DINNER
12 oz. **Chocolate Peanut Butter Banana Smoothie** (see recipe in Week 1, Thurs.), 1 granola or energy bar	1 c. Leftover **Bulgur Wheat Tabouli** (see recipe in Week 4, Wed.) and 2 **Easy Falafel Patties** (see recipe in Week 4, Wed.), 1 c. orange juice	200 calories of whole grain crackers with ½ c. of vegetable salsa or guacamole	Veggie burger with tomato, lettuce, and avocado, 4 oz. **Baked Sweet Potato Fries**, 1 c. almond milk

BAKED SWEET POTATO FRIES

Serves 3

Brown sugar adds a sweet touch to these yummy sweet potato fries. If you like your fries with a kick, add some crushed red pepper flakes or a dash of cayenne pepper to the mix.

2 large sweet potatoes, sliced into fries
2 T. olive oil
¼ t. garlic powder

½ t. paprika
½ t. brown sugar
½ t. chili powder
¼ t. sea salt

1. Preheat oven to 400°F.
2. Spread sweet potatoes on a large baking sheet and drizzle with olive oil, tossing gently to coat.
3. In a small bowl, combine remaining ingredients. Sprinkle over potatoes, coating evenly and tossing as needed.
4. Bake for 10 minutes, turning once. Sprinkle with sea salt.

PER SERVING Calories **161** Fat **9G** Protein **2G** Sodium **255MG** Fiber **3G** Carbohydrates **19G** Sugar **4G** Zinc **0MG** Calcium **29MG** Iron **1MG** Vit. D **0MCG** Vit. B$_{12}$ **0MCG**

THE MANY TEXTURES OF TOFU

Freeze firm or extra-firm tofu for an even meatier and chewier texture, which some people prefer, and which makes it even more absorbent of marinates and sauces. If you're looking for a tofu great in soups, try soft tofu. After pressing your tofu, stick it in the freezer until solid and thaw just before using. If you don't use the whole block, cover any leftover bits of uncooked tofu with water in a sealed container and stick it in the refrigerator.

What I Ate

DATE [ ] | [ ] | [ ]

TIME	FOOD ITEM	AMOUNT	CALORIES	FAT	CARBS	FIBER	PROTEIN
		TOTAL					

Today's Vegan Plate

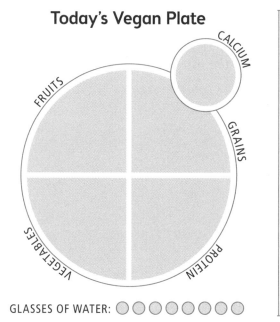

CALCIUM

FRUITS

GRAINS

VEGETABLES

PROTEIN

GLASSES OF WATER: ○ ○ ○ ○ ○ ○ ○ ○

Thoughts about Today

MENU

BREAKFAST	LUNCH	SNACK	DINNER
¾ c. Maple Cinnamon Breakfast Quinoa Bowl, 1 banana	Vegan grilled cheese sandwich on 2 slices whole grain bread with 2 (1-oz.) slices vegan cheese (try Daiya's dairy-free cheese slices or Field Roast's Chao slices), 1 c. tomato soup, 1 apple	1 c. popcorn with 16g nutritional yeast, 1 c. orange juice	1 c. Black Bean and Barley Taco Salad

MAPLE CINNAMON BREAKFAST QUINOA BOWL

Serves 2

Quinoa is a filling and healthy breakfast and has more protein than regular oatmeal. This is a deliciously sweet and energizing way to kick off your day.

1 c. quinoa
2–2½ c. water
1 t. vegan margarine
⅔ c. unsweetended soy milk

½ t. cinnamon
2 T. maple syrup
2 T. raisins
2 medium bananas, sliced

1. Heat quinoa and water in a small saucepan and bring to a boil. Reduce to a simmer and allow to cook, covered, for 15 minutes until liquid is absorbed.
2. Remove from heat and fluff quinoa with a fork. Cover, and allow to sit for 5 minutes.
3. Stir in margarine and soy milk, then the remaining ingredients.

PER SERVING Calories 546 Fat 9G Protein 16G Sodium 57MG Fiber 10G Carbohydrates 105G Sugar 35G Zinc 3MG Calcium 178MG Iron 5MG Vit. D 0MG Vit. B$_{12}$ 1MG

QUINOA FOR BREAKFAST

If you discover you like eating quinoa for breakfast, try quinoa flakes instead of whole quinoa. The flakes are quicker to cook but provide the same protein and amino acids that make quinoa such a great choice for vegans. Also, quinoa flour is great in pancakes, waffles, and muffins!

BLACK BEAN AND BARLEY TACO SALAD

Serves 3

Adding barley to a taco salad gives a bit of a whole grain and fiber boost to this low-fat recipe.

1 (15-oz.) can black beans, drained
½ t. cumin
½ t. dried oregano
2 T. lime juice
1 t. hot chili sauce

1 c. cooked barley
1 medium head iceberg lettuce, shredded
¾ c. salsa
1 oz. handful tortilla chips, crumbled
2 T. vegan Italian dressing

1. Mash together beans, cumin, oregano, lime juice, and hot sauce until beans are mostly mashed, then combine with barley.
2. Layer lettuce with beans and barley, and top with salsa and tortilla chips. Drizzle with Italian dressing.

PER SERVING Calories 300 Fat 7G Protein 11G Sodium 835MG Fiber 11G Carbohydrates 52G Sugar 7G Zinc 2MG Calcium 135MG Iron 3MG Vit. D 0MCG Vit. B$_{12}$ 0MCG

What I Ate

DATE ⬚ | ⬚ | ⬚

TIME	FOOD ITEM	AMOUNT	CALORIES	FAT	CARBS	FIBER	PROTEIN
	TOTAL						

Today's Vegan Plate

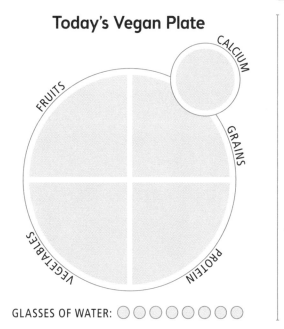

GLASSES OF WATER: ○○○○○○○○

Thoughts about Today

MENU

BREAKFAST	LUNCH	SNACK	DINNER
1 c. instant Cream of Wheat with 1 banana, sliced; 1 c. soy hot chocolate	Quesadilla with 2 (1-oz.) slices vegan cheese, 2 oz. chicken substitute, ¼ c. broccoli, and ½ c. black beans	½ (3") bagel with 1 T. hummus, 1 c. orange juice	½ c. **Lentil and Rice Loaf**, 1 c. vegan mashed potatoes, 1 ear corn on the cob

LENTIL AND RICE LOAF

Serves 8

Made from two of the cheapest ingredients on the planet, this one is a great filler for families on a budget. Use poultry seasoning in place of the individual herbs, if you prefer.

3 cloves garlic, minced	¼ c. unsweetened applesauce
1 large onion, diced	½ t. dried parsley
2 T. olive oil	½ t. dried thyme
3½ c. cooked lentils	½ t. dried oregano
2¼ c. cooked rice	¼ t. dried sage
⅓ c. plus 3 T. ketchup, divided	¾ t. salt
2 T. all-purpose flour	½ t. black pepper

1. Preheat oven to 350°F.
2. Sauté garlic and onion in oil until onion is soft and clear, about 3–4 minutes.
3. In a large bowl, use a fork or a potato masher to mash lentils until about ⅔ mashed.
4. Add garlic and onions, rice, ⅓ cup ketchup, and flour and combine well, then add applesauce and remaining ingredients, mashing to combine.
5. Gently press the mixture into a lightly greased loaf pan. Drizzle the remaining 3 T. ketchup on top.
6. Bake for 60 minutes. Allow to cool at least 10 minutes before serving, as loaf will firm slightly as it cools.

PER SERVING Calories **235** Fat **4G** Protein **10G** Sodium **586MG** Fiber **8G** Carbohydrates **41G** Sugar **7G** Zinc **1MG** Calcium **32MG** Iron **4MG** Vit. D **0MCG** Vit. B$_{12}$ **0MCG**

FOR A PERFECT LENTIL LOAF...

Cook the rice and lentils in vegetable broth and add a bay leaf for maximum flavor. Overcook the lentils a bit so they'll be soft and mash easily. To avoid a mushy loaf, allow both the rice and lentils to cool completely before making your loaf, as they'll be drier that way. Finally, smother the top with loads of ketchup—that's the best part!

What I Ate

DATE [   ] | [   ] | [   ]

TIME	FOOD ITEM	AMOUNT	CALORIES	FAT	CARBS	FIBER	PROTEIN
		TOTAL					

Today's Vegan Plate

FRUITS · CALCIUM · GRAINS · VEGETABLES · PROTEIN

GLASSES OF WATER: ○○○○○○○○

Thoughts about Today

MENU

BREAKFAST	LUNCH	SNACK	DINNER
1 avocado, mashed, on 2 slices whole grain toast with sea salt sprinkled on top, 1 apple	¾ c. Mediterranean Quinoa Pilaf, 1 c. broccoli	1 c. edamame, 1 c. almond milk	Takeout cheeseless pizza with extra vegetables (about 400 calories); side green salad with 2 c. romaine lettuce, 1 tomato, and 1 diced cucumber, and 2 T. Goddess Dressing (see recipe in Week 1, Mon.)

MEDITERRANEAN QUINOA PILAF

Serves 4

Inspired by the flavors of the Mediterranean, bring this vibrant whole grain entrée to a vegan potluck and watch it magically disappear.

1½ c. quinoa
3 c. vegetable broth
3 T. balsamic vinegar
2 T. olive oil
1 T. lemon juice
⅓ t. Himalayan salt

½ c. sun-dried tomatoes, chopped
½ c. artichoke hearts, chopped
½ c. black or kalamata olives, sliced

1. In a large skillet or saucepan, bring quinoa and vegetable broth to a boil, then reduce to a simmer. Cover, and allow quinoa to cook until liquid is absorbed, about 15 minutes. Remove from heat, fluff quinoa with a fork, and allow to stand another 5 minutes.
2. Stir in balsamic vinegar, olive oil, lemon juice, and salt, then add remaining ingredients, gently tossing to combine. Serve hot.

PER SERVING Calories **366** Fat **13G** Protein **11G** Sodium **885MG** Fiber **5G** Carbohydrates **51G** Sugar **7G** Zinc **2MG** Calcium **46MG** Iron **4MG** Vit. D **0MCG** Vit. B$_{12}$ **0MCG**

WHAT'S A PIZZA WITHOUT CHEESE?

More and more pizzerias offer a vegan cheese option these days, but cheeseless pizza is just as delicious. When ordering out, fill your pizza with tons of extra toppings—try olives, whole roasted garlic, mushrooms, pineapple, or even broccoli—and sprinkle it with nutritional yeast if you want that cheesy flavor, or try a vegan ranch dressing to dip it in. If you're not sure where to order a vegan pizza, chains such as Mellow Mushroom, Blaze Pizza, and MOD Pizza all offer vegan-friendly options. Enjoy a night away from the kitchen, and save some leftovers for tomorrow!

What I Ate

DATE [　　　] | [　　　] | [　　　]

TIME	FOOD ITEM	AMOUNT	CALORIES	FAT	CARBS	FIBER	PROTEIN
	TOTAL						

Today's Vegan Plate

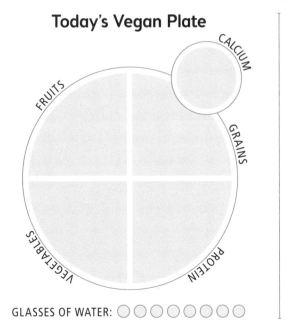

CALCIUM

FRUITS

GRAINS

VEGETABLES

PROTEIN

GLASSES OF WATER: ○○○○○○○○

Thoughts about Today

REVIEW

I FEEL:

_____

_____

_____

_____

MY GREATEST FOOD DISCOVERY THIS WEEK WAS:

_____

_____

_____

_____

THIS WEEK'S BIGGEST VEGAN CHALLENGE WAS:

_____

_____

_____

_____

NEW FOOD I'D LIKE TO TRY:

_____

_____

_____

_____

WHEN I LOOK BACK AT THIS WEEK, I MOST WANT TO REMEMBER:

_____

_____

_____

_____

HOW ARE YOU PROGRESSING TOWARD YOUR GOALS?

_____

_____

_____

_____

WEEK 5

You've been vegan a full month now—congratulations! Most of your physical cravings will have subsided by now. Of course, living in a world full of meat eaters, you're still going to be reminded of animal products, and you may still experience some emotional longing for non-vegan foods, but your tastes have significantly changed by now, and you're probably eating a more varied diet than you ever thought was possible! Keep it up!

If anyone tells you a vegan diet is boring and bland, you'll certainly be proving them wrong this week. It's time to invite friends over to test out your cooking! We'll focus on exploring different palettes of spices and ingredients from around the world, while still keeping the meals simple enough for a busy week.

Two ingredients may be new to you this week: TVP (textured vegetable protein) and tempeh. These are both commonly found soy-based meat substitutes that will soon become regular staples in your kitchen. Look for tempeh in the refrigerated section of your regular grocery store, and TVP is usually found among packaged dry foods in natural foods stores. Larger grocers may sell it in the bulk bins, as well. It may look funny, but don't worry, it's delicious when prepared properly!

MENU

BREAKFAST	LUNCH	SNACK	DINNER
1 c. instant grits with 1 (1-oz.) slice vegan cheese, 1 c. unsweetened applesauce	¾ c. leftover Mediterranean Quinoa Pilaf (see recipe in Week 4, Sun.)	Mixed fruit salad with ½ apple, ½ banana, ½ c. strawberries, and ½ c. pineapple; 1 oz. peanuts	2 c. Ten-Minute Chili topped with 1 (1-oz.) slice vegan cheese, ½ c. Crispy Tempeh Fries

TEN-MINUTE CHILI

Serves 4

No time? No problem! This is a quick and easy way to get some vegetables and protein on the table with no hassle. Instead of a beef crumble alternative, you could toss in a handful of TVP flakes, if you'd like, or any other mock meat you happen to have on hand.

1 (12-oz.) jar salsa
1 (14-oz.) can diced tomatoes
2 (14-oz.) cans kidney beans or black beans, drained
1½ c. frozen vegetables

1 (10-oz.) bag of beef crumble alternative, such as from Beyond Meat
2 T. chili powder
1 t. cumin
½ c. water

In a large pot, combine all ingredients together. Simmer for 10 minutes, stirring frequently.

PER SERVING Calories 368 Fat 7G Protein 31G Sodium 1,652MG Fiber 14G Carbohydrates 50G Sugar 14G Zinc 2MG Calcium 179MG Iron 8MG Vit. D 0MCG Vit. B$_{12}$ 0MCG

CRISPY TEMPEH FRIES

Serves 2

Frying these tempeh sticks twice makes them extracrispy and extradelicious.

1 (8-oz.) package tempeh
2 c. water for boiling
½ t. salt
½ t. garlic powder

1 t. onion powder
2½ t. olive oil for frying
½ t. seasoning salt

1. Slice tempeh into thin strips. Simmer tempeh, covered, in 1" water for 10 minutes. Drain.
2. While tempeh is still moist, sprinkle with salt, garlic powder, and onion powder.
3. Heat oil and fry tempeh for 5–6 minutes until crispy and browned. Place tempeh on paper towels and allow to cool for at least 30 minutes.
4. Reheat oil and fry again for another 4–5 minutes. Season with seasoning salt while still warm.

PER SERVING Calories 279 Fat 18G Protein 24G Sodium 613MG Fiber 0G Carbohydrates 11G Sugar 0G Zinc 1MG Calcium 133MG Iron 3MG Vit. D 0MCG Vit. B$_{12}$ 0MCG

TEMPEH 101

Most tempeh recipes will turn out better if your tempeh is simmered in a bit of water or vegetable broth first. This improves the digestibility of the tempeh, softens it up, decreases the cooking time, and, if you add some seasonings such as soy sauce, garlic powder, or some herbs, will increase the flavor as well.

What I Ate

DATE [ ] | [ ] | [ ]

TIME	FOOD ITEM	AMOUNT	CALORIES	FAT	CARBS	FIBER	PROTEIN
TOTAL							

Today's Vegan Plate

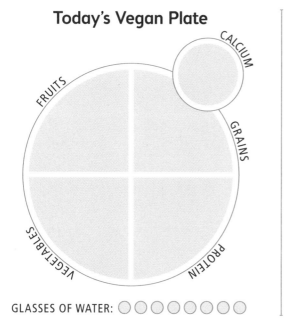

GLASSES OF WATER: ○ ○ ○ ○ ○ ○ ○ ○

Thoughts about Today

BREAKFAST	LUNCH	SNACK	DINNER
1 T. almond butter and 1 banana, sliced, on 2 slices whole wheat bread or bagel; 1 c. soy hot chocolate	Veggie hot dogs (try Lightlife or Tofurky hot dogs) with vegetarian baked beans (or other toppings of your preference) on top, 1 c. diced pineapple	½ c. leftover **Crispy Tempeh Fries** (see recipe in Week 5, Mon.) dipped in ¼ c. **Basic Vegetable Marinara** (see recipe in Week 1, Mon.)	1½ c. **Pineapple Cauliflower Curry** with 1 c. brown rice and 1 c. orange juice

PINEAPPLE CAULIFLOWER CURRY

Serves 4

To save time chopping, substitute a bag of mixed frozen vegetables or toss in some leftover cooked potatoes to this tropical *Instagram*-worthy yellow curry recipe. Serve hot over rice or another whole grain.

¾ c. vegetable broth
1 c. regular coconut milk, unsweetended
1½ c. green peas
1 medium head cauliflower, chopped
2 medium carrots, chopped small
2 t. fresh ginger, minced
3 cloves garlic, minced
2 t. curry powder
½ t. turmeric
1 t. brown sugar
¼ t. salt
¼ t. nutmeg
1 c. diced pineapple
2 T. chopped fresh cilantro

1. Whisk together vegetable broth and coconut milk in a large saucepan.
2. Add remaining ingredients except pineapple and cilantro, stirring well to combine. Bring to a slow simmer, cover, and cook for 8–10 minutes, stirring occasionally. Add pineapple and heat for 2 more minutes.
3. Top with fresh cilantro.

PER SERVING Calories **136** Fat **2G** Protein **7G** Sodium **375MG** Fiber **7G** Carbohydrates **26G** Sugar **12G** Zinc **1MG** Calcium **98MG** Iron **2MG** Vit. D **1MCG** Vit. B$_{12}$ **1MCG**

MAKE YOUR OWN NUT BUTTER

Nut butters are often expensive to purchase, but they are so easy to make at home! You can use this method to make just about any kind of nut butter you like. Try making almond, walnut, or macadamia nut butter for a delicious alternative to store-bought peanut butter. Just process the nuts, then add oil and salt to get a taste and consistency that you like. Roasted nuts work best, so heat them in the oven at 400°F for 6–8 minutes or toast them in a dry skillet on the stove top for a few minutes.

What I Ate

DATE ____ | ____ | ____

TIME	FOOD ITEM	AMOUNT	CALORIES	FAT	CARBS	FIBER	PROTEIN
		TOTAL					

Today's Vegan Plate

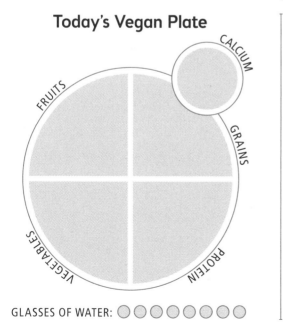

GLASSES OF WATER: ○○○○○○○○

Thoughts about Today

MENU

BREAKFAST	LUNCH	SNACK	DINNER
Cream cheese tortilla wrap with 1 T. vegan cream cheese, ½ apple, sliced, 1 oz. walnuts, 1 oz. raisins, and ¼ t. cinnamon on a flour tortilla	Baked potato with ½ c. black beans, ¼ c. salsa, and 1 (1-oz.) slice vegan cheese; 1 c. tomato juice (no salt added)	1 (6") pita with 2 T. hummus	1 taco with TVP Taco "Meat"; side green salad with 2 c. romaine lettuce or greens of your choice, 1 tomato, 1 diced cucumber, and 2 T. Goddess Dressing (see recipe in Week 1, Mon.); 1 c. broccoli with 16g nutritional yeast

TVP TACO "MEAT"

Serves 6

Whip up this meaty and economical taco filling in just a few minutes using prepared salsa, and have diners fill their own tacos how they like. Nondairy sour cream, vegan cheese, fresh tomatoes, shredded lettuce, avocados, and extra hot sauce are a must.

2 c. TVP flakes	2 T. olive oil
2 c. hot water	2 t. chili powder
1 medium yellow onion, diced	1 t. cumin
½ medium yellow bell pepper, diced	½ c. salsa
	½ t. hot sauce, or to taste
½ medium green bell pepper, diced	6 large flour tortillas

1. Combine TVP with hot water and allow to sit for 5–10 minutes to reconstitute. Drain.
2. In a large skillet, heat onion and bell peppers in olive oil. Add TVP, chili powder, and cumin. Cook, stirring frequently, for 4–5 minutes, or until peppers and onion are soft.
3. Add salsa and hot sauce, stirring to combine. Remove from heat.
4. Wrap TVP mixture in flour tortillas and serve with taco fillings.

PER SERVING Calories 389 Fat 10G Protein 23G Sodium 712MG Fiber 9G Carbohydrates 50G Sugar 9G Zinc 1MG Calcium 227MG Iron 7MG Vit. D 0MCG Vit. B$_{12}$ 0MCG

TEXTURED VEGETABLE PROTEIN

TVP is inexpensive and has such a meaty texture that many budget-conscious non-vegan cooks use it to stretch their dollar, adding it to homemade burgers and meatloaves. For the best deal, buy it in bulk. TVP is usually found in small crumbles, but some stores also sell it in strips or chunks.

What I Ate

DATE [ ] | [ ] | [ ]

TIME	FOOD ITEM	AMOUNT	CALORIES	FAT	CARBS	FIBER	PROTEIN
	TOTAL						

Today's Vegan Plate

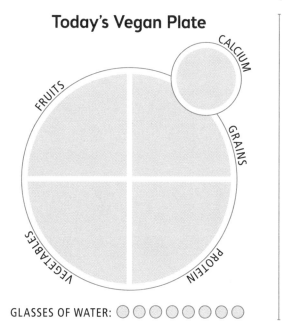

GLASSES OF WATER: ◯◯◯◯◯◯◯◯

Thoughts about Today

MENU

BREAKFAST	LUNCH	SNACK	DINNER
1 c. whole grain cereal, 1 c. hemp milk	½ c. **Tempeh Dill "Chicken" Salad** on 2 slices whole grain bread with ¼ tomato, sliced, and ¼ c. iceberg lettuce	1 c. soy yogurt with ⅓ c. granola	1 c. **Thai Tom Kha Coconut Soup** with ½ c. brown rice

TEMPEH DILL "CHICKEN" SALAD

Serves 4

For curried chicken salad, omit the dill and add ½ t. curry powder and a dash of cayenne and black pepper.

1 (8-oz.) package tempeh, diced small	1 t. Dijon mustard
Water for boiling	2 T. sweet pickle relish
3 T. vegan mayonnaise	½ c. green peas
2 t. lemon juice	2 stalks celery, diced small
½ t. garlic powder	1 T. chopped fresh dill

1. Cover tempeh with water and simmer for 10 minutes until tempeh is soft. Drain and allow to cool completely.
2. Whisk together mayonnaise, lemon juice, garlic powder, mustard, and relish.
3. Combine tempeh, mayonnaise mixture, peas, celery, and dill, and gently toss to combine.
4. Chill for at least 1 hour before serving to allow flavors to combine.

PER SERVING Calories **204** Fat **14G** Protein **13G** Sodium **185MG** Fiber **1G** Carbohydrates **10G** Sugar **3G** Zinc **1MG** Calcium **75MG** Iron **2MG** Vit. D **0MCG** Vit. B$_{12}$ **0MCG**

THAI TOM KHA COCONUT SOUP

Serves 5

Pair this soup with brown rice for a satisfying meal. Use lime and ginger if you can't find lemongrass or galangal.

1 (14-oz.) can regular coconut milk, unsweetened	2 small chilies, chopped
	½ t. red pepper flakes
2 c. vegetable broth	1 medium onion, chopped
1 T. soy sauce	2 medium tomatoes, chopped
3 cloves garlic, minced	
5 slices fresh ginger or galangal	1 medium carrot, sliced thin
1 stalk lemongrass, chopped	½ c. sliced shiitake mushrooms
1 T. lime juice	¼ c. chopped fresh cilantro

1. Combine coconut milk and vegetable broth over medium-low heat. Add soy sauce, garlic, ginger, lemongrass, lime juice, chilies, and red pepper flakes. Heat, but do not boil.
2. When broth is hot, add onion, tomatoes, carrot, and mushrooms. Cover and cook on low heat for 10–15 minutes.
3. Remove from heat and top with chopped fresh cilantro.

PER SERVING Calories **51G** Fat **2G** Protein **2G** Sodium **455MG** Fiber **2G** Carbohydrates **8G** Sugar **4G** Zinc **0MG** Calcium **51MG** Iron **1MG** Vit. D **1MCG** Vit. B$_{12}$ **1MCG**

TAKE CARE OF YOUR HERBS

Make fresh herbs last longer by giving them a quick rinse. Then wrap your lightly damp herbs in a paper towel and place in a ziptop bag. Store in your refrigerator's crisper. They'll keep about ten days this way.

What I Ate

DATE ⬚ | ⬚ | ⬚

TIME	FOOD ITEM	AMOUNT	CALORIES	FAT	CARBS	FIBER	PROTEIN
		TOTAL					

Today's Vegan Plate

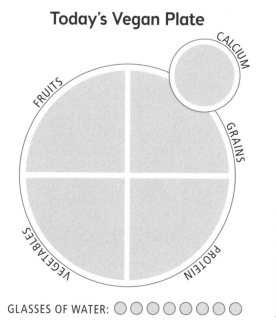

GLASSES OF WATER: ◯◯◯◯◯◯◯◯

Thoughts about Today

MENU

BREAKFAST	LUNCH	SNACK	DINNER
2 c. **Strawberry Protein Smoothie** (see recipe in Week 2, Tues.)	Bean burrito with 1 large flour tortilla with 1 c. refried beans, ¼ tomato (sliced), ¼ c. spinach, ¼ c. rice, and 1 diced avocado	Mixed fruit salad with ½ apple, ½ banana, ½ c. strawberries, and ½ c. pineapple; 1 granola or energy bar	1 c. **Saucy Chinese Veggies with Tempeh** with rice noodles, 1 c. orange juice

SAUCY CHINESE VEGGIES WITH TEMPEH

Serves 5

This is a simple and basic stir-fry recipe with Asian ingredients and suitable for a main dish. Serve over noodles or rice. Swap in 1 cup chopped seitan if you prefer. If you don't have water chestnuts or bamboo shoots, simply omit them.

1½ c. vegetable broth
3 T. soy sauce
1 T. rice vinegar
1 t. minced ginger
1 t. sugar
1 (8-oz.) block tempeh, cubed
2 T. olive oil
1 medium red bell pepper, chopped

1 c. snow peas
¾ pound of broccoli florets
½ c. sliced water chestnuts
¼ c. sliced bamboo shoots
2 scallions, sliced
1 T. cornstarch

1. In a small bowl, whisk together vegetable broth, soy sauce, rice vinegar, ginger, and sugar.
2. In a large skillet, brown tempeh or seitan in olive oil on all sides, about 3–4 minutes.
3. Add bell pepper, snow peas, broccoli, water chestnuts, bamboo shoots, and scallions, and heat just until vegetables are almost soft, about 2–3 minutes, stirring constantly.
4. Reduce heat and add vegetable broth mixture. Whisk in cornstarch. Bring to a slow simmer and cook until thickened, stirring to prevent lumps.

PER SERVING Calories **204** Fat **11G** Protein **13G** Sodium **751MG** Fiber **3G** Carbohydrates **17G** Sugar **5G** Zinc **1G** Calcium **108MG** Iron **3MG** Vit. D **0MCG** Vit. B₁₂ **0MCG**

THAT'S VEE-GUN, NOT VAY-GUN

Donald Watson, a British farmer, first created the word *vegan* (the beginning and end of "vegetarian," he reasoned) in 1944, when he founded the Vegan Society in England. He led a mostly quiet life, shunning any fame associated with his revolutionary ideas. At the time of his death at ninety-five years old, he had been vegan for sixty-one years, and vegetarian for more than eighty.

What I Ate

DATE ____ | ____ | ____

TIME	FOOD ITEM	AMOUNT	CALORIES	FAT	CARBS	FIBER	PROTEIN
	TOTAL						

Today's Vegan Plate

Thoughts about Today

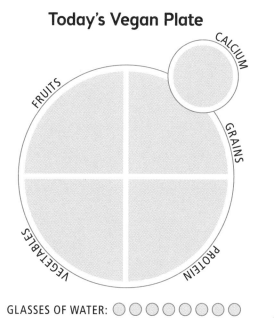

GLASSES OF WATER: ○○○○○○○○

MENU

BREAKFAST	LUNCH	SNACK	DINNER
3 oz. **Basic Creamy Polenta**, 1 vegan sausage patty, 1 c. orange juice	Vegan Caesar salad with 2 c. romaine lettuce, 3 oz. vegan chicken, and store-bought dressing of your choice; 1 small steamed sweet potato; 1 c. orange juice	2 oz. **Sugar-Free No-Bake Cocoa Balls**	1 c. **Lentil Vegetable Soup**; 1 slice whole grain toast; 1 c. oven-roasted butternut squash; 1 c. collard greens sautéed with ½ T. olive oil, 1 minced clove garlic, and dash sea salt

BASIC CREAMY POLENTA

Serves 4

Top this dish with mixed berries for a sweet treat.

6½ c. water	**1½ t. garlic powder**
2 c. cornmeal (polenta)	**¼ c. nutritional yeast**
3 T. vegan margarine	**½ t. salt**

1. Bring water to a boil, then slowly add polenta, stirring to combine.
2. Reduce heat to low, and cook for 20 minutes, stirring frequently. Polenta is done when it is thick and sticky.
3. Stir in margarine, garlic powder, nutritional yeast, and salt.

PER SERVING Calories **380** Fat **10G** Protein **7G** Sodium **393MG** Fiber **4G** Carbohydrates **64G** Sugar **1G** Zinc **1MG** Calcium **4MG** Iron **4MG** Vit. D **0MCG** Vit. B$_{12}$ **0MCG**

SUGAR-FREE NO-BAKE COCOA BALLS

Serves 5

If you have a sweet tooth, these cocoa balls will satisfy it—while providing fiber and protein.

1 c. chopped pitted dates	**¼ c. cocoa powder**
Water for soaking	**1 T. peanut butter**
1 c. walnuts or cashews	**¼ c. coconut flakes**

1. Cover dates in water and soak for about 10 minutes until softened. Drain.
2. Process dates, nuts, cocoa powder, peanut butter, and coconut flakes in a food processor until coarse.
3. Shape into balls and place in freezer for 30 minutes, until somewhat firm.

PER SERVING Calories **218** Fat **19G** Protein **5G** Sodium **3MG** Fiber **4G** Carbohydrates **13G** Sugar **7G** Zinc **1MG** Calcium **36MG** Iron **2MG** Vit. D **0MCG** Vit. B$_{12}$ **0MCG**

LENTIL VEGETABLE SOUP

Serves 4

This hearty soup is perfect for using up leftover vegetables.

1 medium onion, diced	**2 medium yellow potatoes, chopped**
2 cloves garlic, minced	**1 c. dry lentils**
2 stalks celery, chopped	**½ t. dried thyme**
1 medium zucchini, diced	**¼ t. dried oregano**
1 medium carrot, chopped	**2 bay leaves**
1 T. olive oil	**1 t. salt**
2 c. water	**1 t. black pepper**
4 c. vegetable broth	**2 c. spinach**
	1 T. fresh lemon juice

1. In a large pot, sauté onion, garlic, celery, zucchini, and carrot in olive oil for 4–5 minutes until onion is soft. Reduce heat and add remaining ingredients, except for spinach and lemon juice.
2. Bring to a slow simmer. Cover and heat until lentils are cooked through, about 45 minutes. Stir in spinach leaves and heat another 5 minutes until spinach has wilted.
3. Remove bay leaves and drizzle with lemon juice just before serving.

PER SERVING Calories **322** Fat **4G** Protein **16G** Sodium **1,280MG** Fiber **8G** Carbohydrates **58G** Sugar **5G** Zinc **2MG** Calcium **74MG** Iron **5MG** Vit. D **0MCG** Vit. B$_{12}$ **0MCG**

What I Ate

DATE ___ | ___ | ___

TIME	FOOD ITEM	AMOUNT	CALORIES	FAT	CARBS	FIBER	PROTEIN
	TOTAL						

Today's Vegan Plate

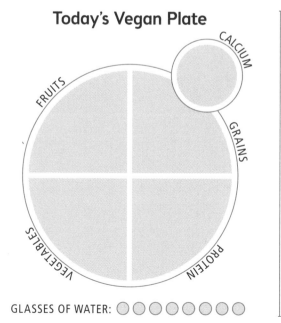

GLASSES OF WATER: ○○○○○○○○

Thoughts about Today

MENU

BREAKFAST	LUNCH	SNACK	DINNER
1 (3") bagel with 1 T. peanut butter and 1 banana, 1 c. plant-based milk	1 c. leftover Lentil Vegetable Soup (see recipe in Week 5, Sat.), 1 slice whole grain toast, 1 c. orange juice	1 c. Crispy Baked Kale Chips, 2 oz. cashews	1 c. Cheesy Macaroni and "Hamburger" Casserole, ½ c. sautéed zucchini

CRISPY BAKED KALE CHIPS

Serves 1

Kale is packed with antioxidants, is a great source of vitamin C and vitamin K, and can help lower cholesterol.

1 large bunch of kale
2 t. olive oil
½ t. garlic salt
1 t. nutritional yeast

1. Preheat oven to 350°F.
2. Chop kale into bite-sized pieces and place in a large bowl. Gently toss together with olive oil and garlic salt.
3. Arrange kale in a single layer on a baking sheet and sprinkle well with nutritional yeast. Bake for 20–25 minutes until nicely crisped.

PER SERVING Calories 218 Fat 11G Protein 10G Sodium 1,275MG Fiber 10G Carbohydrates 27G Sugar 6G Zinc 1MG Calcium 344MG Iron 4MG Vit. D 0MCG Vit. B$_{12}$ 0MCG

CHEESY MACARONI AND "HAMBURGER" CASSEROLE

Serves 5

This casserole evokes flavors of a traditional comfort food, but veganized!

1 (12-oz.) bag macaroni noodles (try Daiya's dairy-free Deluxe Cheddar Style Cheezy Mac or Upton's Naturals Ch'eesy Mac)
1 (12-oz.) package vegan beef crumbles
1 medium tomato, diced
1 T. olive oil
1 t. chili powder
1 c. unsweetened soy milk
2 T. vegan margarine
2 T. all-purpose flour
1 t. garlic powder
1 t. onion powder
¼ c. nutritional yeast
1 t. salt
1 t. black pepper

1. Prepare macaroni noodles according to package instructions.
2. Sauté beef crumbles and tomato in olive oil until "hamburger" is lightly browned, and season with chili powder.
3. In a separate small skillet, melt together soy milk and margarine over low heat until well mixed. Stir in flour and heat until thickened, then stir in garlic powder, onion powder, and nutritional yeast and remove from heat.
4. Combine macaroni, beef crumbles, tomato, and sauce, gently tossing to coat.
5. Season with salt and pepper, and allow to cool slightly before serving to allow ingredients to combine.

PER SERVING Calories 312 Fat 13G Protein 7G Sodium 955MG Fiber 3G Carbohydrates 41G Sugar 3G Zinc 1MG Calcium 156MG Iron 2MG Vit. D 0MCG Vit. B$_{12}$ 4MCG

MOCK GROUND BEEF

Vegan ground beef is tasty and can be used in the same way you would use regular ground beef. Brown it in a bit of oil in a sauté pan and add it to casseroles, pasta sauces, or use as an enchilada or burrito filling.

What I Ate

DATE [   ] | [   ] | [   ]

TIME	FOOD ITEM	AMOUNT	CALORIES	FAT	CARBS	FIBER	PROTEIN
		TOTAL					

Today's Vegan Plate

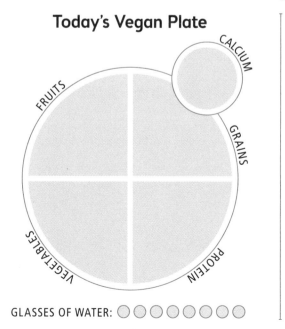

FRUITS

CALCIUM

GRAINS

VEGETABLES

PROTEIN

GLASSES OF WATER: ○○○○○○○○

Thoughts about Today

REVIEW

I FEEL:

_____

_____

_____

_____

MY GREATEST FOOD DISCOVERY THIS WEEK WAS:

_____

_____

_____

_____

THIS WEEK'S BIGGEST VEGAN CHALLENGE WAS:

_____

_____

_____

_____

NEW FOOD I'D LIKE TO TRY:

_____

_____

_____

_____

WHEN I LOOK BACK AT THIS WEEK, I MOST WANT TO REMEMBER:

_____

_____

_____

_____

HOW ARE YOU PROGRESSING TOWARD YOUR GOALS?

_____

_____

_____

_____

WEEK 6

By now, your body is mostly done adjusting to your new diet, and you probably haven't been experiencing any withdrawal symptoms for a while. In short, you should be feeling great this week! Your body is getting used to this new way of eating, and you could probably find your way around the grocery store (and your kitchen) in the dark.

If you've never tried seitan (say-tan), or tried making it yourself, now's your chance. The food originated in China and Japan more than one thousand years ago. When made from scratch, seitan is the most affordable of all the meat substitutes. It's available store-bought, but making it at home will help your pocketbook immensely. Tofu, tempeh, seitan, and other store-bought mock meats are largely interchangeable, so if you find you like one more than the other, feel free to change it up. They're all great sources of protein. Before you decide that you don't like one of these substitutes, be sure to try it not just once, but twice, two different ways. Look for store-bought seitan (also called wheat gluten) in the refrigerated section of your natural foods store.

The menu plans call for a bit of experimentation with vegan baking this week and next, so make sure you've got a good egg substitute on hand. If you enjoy baking and don't want to stop with just banana bread and muffins, try a homemade batch of vegan cookies!

BREAKFAST	LUNCH	SNACK	DINNER
1 c. **Chili Masala Tofu Scramble** (see recipe in Week 2, Sat.), 1 c. fresh strawberries	Hummus and roasted red pepper sandwich with 2 T. hummus, 1 oz. roasted red pepper, 1 sliced avocado, ¼ c. diced tomato, and ½ c. sprouts on 2 slices of whole wheat bread; green salad; 2 oz. cashews	200 calories of whole grain chips with ½ c. salsa, 1 apple or 1 sliced mango	1 c. **Breaded Eggplant "Parmesan"**

BREADED EGGPLANT "PARMESAN"

Serves 4

Slowly baking these breaded eggplant cutlets brings out the best flavor, but they can also be panfried in a bit of oil.

1 medium eggplant	4 T. unsweetened apple-
½ t. salt	sauce (for replacement
¾ c. all-purpose flour	of 2 eggs)
1 t. garlic powder	1½ c. bread crumbs
⅔ c. unsweetened soy milk	2 T. Italian seasonings
	¼ c. nutritional yeast
	1½ c. Basic Vegetable Marinara (see recipe in Week 1, Mon.)

1. Slice eggplant into ¾"-thick slices and sprinkle with salt. Allow to sit for 10 minutes. Gently pat dry to remove extra moisture.
2. In a shallow bowl or pie tin, combine flour and garlic powder. In a separate bowl, whisk together soy milk and applacesauce. In a third bowl, combine bread crumbs, Italian seasonings, and nutritional yeast.
3. Coat each eggplant slice with flour, then dip in the soy milk mixture, then coat with the bread crumb mixture and place in a greased casserole dish.
4. Bake for 20–25 minutes, then top with marinara sauce, and return to oven until sauce is hot, about 5 minutes.

PER SERVING Calories **386** Fat **6G** Protein **14G** Sodium **859MG** Fiber **10G** Carbohydrates **70G** Sugar **15G** Zinc **2MG** Calcium **155MG** Iron **6MG** Vit. D **0MCG** Vit. B$_{12}$ **5MCG**

ROASTED RED PEPPERS

Sure, you can buy them from a jar, but it's also easy to roast your own. Here's how: Fire up your oven to 450°F (or use the broiler setting) and drizzle a few whole peppers with olive oil. Bake for 30 minutes, turning over once. Direct heat will also work; if you have a gas stove hold the peppers with tongs over the flame until lightly charred. Once they're cool, removing the skin is optional. Add your roasted red peppers to homemade hummus, sandwiches and wraps, pasta sauces, and salads for a gourmet touch. Voilà!

What I Ate

DATE [   ] | [   ] | [   ]

TIME	FOOD ITEM	AMOUNT	CALORIES	FAT	CARBS	FIBER	PROTEIN
		TOTAL					

Today's Vegan Plate

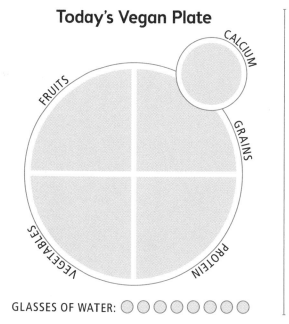

CALCIUM

FRUITS

GRAINS

VEGETABLES

PROTEIN

GLASSES OF WATER: ○○○○○○○○○

Thoughts about Today

MENU

BREAKFAST	LUNCH	SNACK	DINNER
1 large flour tortilla breakfast wrap with 1 T. almond butter and ⅓ c. granola, 1 c. orange juice	1 c. leftover **Breaded Eggplant "Parmesan"** (see recipe in Week 6, Mon.); Greek spinach salad with 2 c. fresh spinach, 1 medium tomato, ½ red bell pepper, 2 T. black olives, ¼ c. chopped artichoke hearts, and 2 T. **Goddess Dressing** (see recipe in Week 1, Mon.)	Mixed vegetables (½ cucumber, 2 oz. baby carrots, ½ c. broccoli) with 2 T. hummus, 1 banana	5 oz. **Seitan Barbecue "Meat,"** 1 sweet potato, 1 ear corn on the cob with 16g nutritional yeast

SEITAN BARBECUE "MEAT"

Serves 6

Sooner or later, all vegans discover the magically delicious combination of seitan and barbecue sauce in some variation of this classic favorite.

1 (12-oz.) package pre-
  pared seitan, chopped
  into thin strips (about
  2 c.)
1 large sweet onion,
  chopped

3 cloves garlic, minced
2 T. olive oil
1 c. barbecue sauce
2 T. water

1. Heat seitan, onion, and garlic in olive oil, stirring frequently until onion is just soft and seitan is lightly browned.
2. Reduce heat to medium low and stir in barbecue sauce and water. Allow to simmer, stirring to coat seitan until most of the liquid has been absorbed, about 10 minutes.

PER SERVING Calories 191 Fat **5G** Protein **11G** Sodium **636MG** Fiber **2G** Carbohydrates **27G** Sugar **17G** Zinc **0MG** Calcium **50MG** Iron **1MG** Vit. D **0MCG** Vit. B$_{12}$ **0MCG**

SAVE THE LEFTOVERS FOR LUNCH TOMORROW

Piled on top of sourdough along with some vegan mayonnaise, lettuce, avocado, and tomato, thinly sliced seitan always makes a perfect sandwich. Melt some vegan cheese for a simple Philly "cheesesteak"–style sandwich, or pile on the vegan Thousand Island and sauerkraut for a seitan Reuben. Seitan is also great grilled, so you can also try grilling tonight's seitan instead of panfrying it.

What I Ate

DATE [   ] | [   ] | [   ]

TIME	FOOD ITEM	AMOUNT	CALORIES	FAT	CARBS	FIBER	PROTEIN
TOTAL							

Today's Vegan Plate

CALCIUM

FRUITS

GRAINS

VEGETABLES

PROTEIN

Thoughts about Today

GLASSES OF WATER: ○○○○○○○○

BREAKFAST	LUNCH	SNACK	DINNER
1 c. oatmeal breakfast bowl with 1 oz. almonds, 1 banana or 1 c. strawberries, and 2 t. maple syrup; 1 c. soy hot chocolate	5 oz. leftover Seitan Barbecue "Meat" (see recipe in Week 6, Tues.) on 2 slices of whole wheat bread, with ¼ tomato (sliced), ¼ c. kale, and 1 T. vegan mayonnaise; 1 apple or 1 c. grapes	½ (3") bagel topped with 2 T. guacamole	1 patty Easy Black Bean Burgers, 2 oz. Breaded Baked Zucchini Chips, 1 c. orange juice

EASY BLACK BEAN BURGERS

Yields 6 patties

Veggie burgers are notorious for falling apart. If you're sick of crumbly burgers, try this simple method for making black bean patties. It's 100 percent guaranteed to stick together.

1 (15-oz.) can black beans, drained
3 T. minced onions
1 t. salt
1½ t. garlic powder
2 t. dried parsley
1 t. chili powder
⅔ c. all-purpose flour
2½ t. olive oil for panfrying

1. Process black beans in a blender or food processor until halfway mashed, or mash with a fork.
2. Add minced onions, salt, garlic powder, parsley, and chili powder, and mash to combine.
3. Add flour, a bit at a time, again mashing together to combine. You may need a little bit more or less than ⅔ cup. Beans should stick together completely.
4. Form into patties and panfry in a bit of oil for 2–3 minutes on each side. Patties will appear to be done on the outside while still a bit mushy on the inside, so fry them a few minutes longer than you think they need.

PER SERVING Calories 126 Fat 3G Protein 5G Sodium 518MG Fiber 3G Carbohydrates 21G Sugar 1G Zinc 0MG Calcium 36MG Iron 1MG Vit. D 0MCG Vit. B$_{12}$ 0MCG

BREADED BAKED ZUCCHINI CHIPS

Serves 4

Looking for a new way to eat zucchini? These tasty chips are perfect for a light snack.

¾ c. fine bread crumbs
½ t. Italian seasoning blend
½ t. garlic powder
¼ t. salt
⅓ c. unsweetened soy milk
2 medium zucchini, sliced into ½"-thick rounds

1. Preheat oven to 475°F and lightly grease a baking sheet.
2. In a large bowl, combine bread crumbs, Italian seasoning, garlic powder, and salt. Place soy milk in a separate small bowl.
3. Gently dip each slice of zucchini into the soy milk, then coat well with bread crumb mix. Arrange breaded zucchini slices on a single layer on baking tray, then bake for 5–10 minutes, or until lightly crisped. Turn zucchini chips over, then bake for another 5 minutes.

PER SERVING Calories 108 Fat 2G Protein 5G Sodium 312MG Fiber 2G Carbohydrates 19G Sugar 4G Zinc 1MG Calcium 62MG Iron 2MG Vit. D 0MCG Vit. B$_{12}$ 0MCG

VEGGIE BURGER TIPS

If you have trouble with your homemade veggie burgers crumbling, try adding egg replacement to bind the ingredients, then chill the mixture before forming into patties. If you are short on time, brands such as Gardein, Field Roast, and Beyond Meat all make plant-based burgers.

What I Ate

DATE ☐ | ☐ | ☐

TIME	FOOD ITEM	AMOUNT	CALORIES	FAT	CARBS	FIBER	PROTEIN
		TOTAL					

Today's Vegan Plate

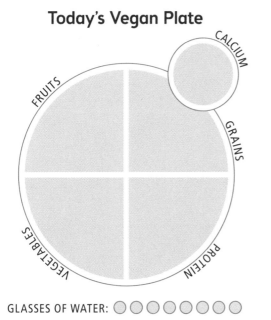

GLASSES OF WATER: ○○○○○○○○

Thoughts about Today

MENU

BREAKFAST	LUNCH	SNACK	DINNER
1 c. **Pumpkin Protein Smoothie** (see recipe in Week 3, Thurs.), 1 banana or 1 c. blueberries, 1 oz. cashews	Vegan deli slices (try Tofurky or Lightlife deli slices) on 2 slices of whole grain bread with 1 tomato slice, ¼ avocado, ½ c. sprouts, and vegan mayonnaise; 1 apple	2 oz. leftover **Breaded Baked Zucchini Chips** (see recipe in Week 6, Wed.)	2 **Fresh Mint Spring Rolls**, ½ c. **Baked Teriyaki Tofu Cubes** (see recipe in Week 3, Fri.)

FRESH MINT SPRING ROLLS

Serves 5

The fresh mint in these rolls is an unexpected delight—it adds a bright flavor and tempers the hot sauce.

1 (3-oz.) package clear bean thread noodles	1 medium carrot, grated
1 c. hot water	10 spring roll wrappers
1 T. soy sauce	Warm water
½ t. powdered ginger	½ medium head green leaf lettuce, chopped
1 t. sesame oil	1 medium cucumber, sliced thin
¼ c. shiitake mushrooms, diced	1 bunch fresh mint

1. Break noodles in half to make smaller pieces, then submerge in 1 cup hot water until soft, about 6–7 minutes. Drain.
2. In a large bowl, toss together hot noodles with soy sauce, ginger, sesame oil, mushrooms, and carrot, tossing well to combine.
3. In a large shallow pan, carefully submerge spring roll wrappers, 1 at a time, in warm water until just barely soft. Remove from water and place a bit of lettuce in the center of the wrapper. Add about 2 T. of noodle mixture, a few slices of cucumber, and place 2 mint leaves on top.
4. Fold the bottom of the wrapper over the filling, fold in each side, then roll.

PER SERVING Calories **154** Fat **1G** Protein **3G** Sodium **369MG** Fiber **2G** Carbohydrates **33G** Sugar **3G** Zinc **0MG** Calcium **49MG** Iron **1MG** Vit. D **0MCG** Vit. B$_{12}$ **0MCG**

HOW TO WRAP SPRING ROLLS

Wrapping spring rolls is a balance between getting them tight enough to hold together, but not so tight that the thin wrappers break! It's like riding a bike: Once you've got it, you've got it, and then spring rolls can be very quick and fun to make. Dip them in store-bought sweet chili sauce, spicy sriracha sauce, Japanese salad dressing, or Chinese hoisin sauce.

What I Ate

DATE [   ] | [   ] | [   ]

TIME	FOOD ITEM	AMOUNT	CALORIES	FAT	CARBS	FIBER	PROTEIN
		TOTAL					

Today's Vegan Plate

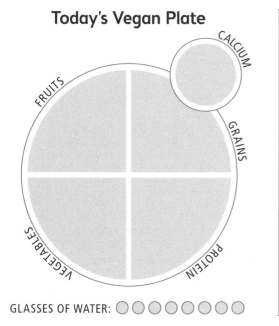

GLASSES OF WATER: ◯◯◯◯◯◯◯◯

Thoughts about Today

MENU

BREAKFAST	LUNCH	SNACK	DINNER
1 c. whole grain cereal with ½ c. cashew milk	Quinoa lunch bowl (1 c. cooked quinoa with 1 c. spinach and 1 c. zucchini, ½ sliced avocado, and ½ c. sunflower seeds)	1 c. edamame	5 oz. **Tofu "Chicken" Nuggets**, 1 ear corn on the cob, 1 medium sweet potato

TOFU "CHICKEN" NUGGETS

Serves 4

Chicken nuggets are a classic favorite for kids and adults alike. Serve these with several different vegan dipping sauces.

- **¼ c. unsweetened soy milk**
- **2 T. mustard**
- **3 T. nutritional yeast**
- **½ c. bread crumbs**
- **½ c. all-purpose flour**
- **1 t. poultry seasoning**
- **1 t. garlic powder**
- **1 t. onion powder**
- **½ t. salt**
- **¼ t. black pepper**
- **1 (14-oz.) block firm or extra-firm tofu, sliced into thin strips**

1. In a large shallow pan, whisk together soy milk, mustard, and nutritional yeast. In a separate bowl, combine bread crumbs with flour, poultry seasoning, garlic powder, onion powder, salt, and pepper.
2. Coat each piece of tofu with the soy milk mixture, then coat well in bread crumbs and flour mixture.
3. Bake in 375°F oven for 20 minutes, turning over once.

PER SERVING Calories **232** Fat **7G** Protein **16G** Sodium **489MG** Fiber **3G** Carbohydrates **27G** Sugar **2G** Zinc **1MG** Calcium **117MG** Iron **3MG** Vit. D **0MCG** Vit. B$_{12}$ **3MCG**

What I Ate

DATE [   ] | [   ] | [   ]

TIME	FOOD ITEM	AMOUNT	CALORIES	FAT	CARBS	FIBER	PROTEIN
	TOTAL						

Today's Vegan Plate

FRUITS
CALCIUM
GRAINS
VEGETABLES
PROTEIN

GLASSES OF WATER: ○○○○○○○○

Thoughts about Today

MENU

BREAKFAST	LUNCH	SNACK	DINNER
2 oz. **Basic Creamy Polenta** (see recipe in Week 5, Sat.) with 2 (1-oz.) slices vegan cheese, ¼ c. black beans, and 2 T. vegetable salsa	1½ c. **Italian White Bean and Fresh Herb Salad** (see recipe in Week 1, Fri.), 1 apple	Mixed fruit salad with ½ apple, ½ banana, ½ c. strawberries, and ½ c. pineapple; 1 granola bar (aim for a fortified bar, with about 150 calories)	5 oz. **Classic Fettuccine Alfredo**; ½ lb. collard greens sautéed with ½ T. olive oil, 1 minced garlic clove, and dash sea salt

CLASSIC FETTUCCINE ALFREDO

Serves 4

This comfort-food favorite will be a surefire winner. If you have any leftovers, reheat them for lunch.

½ c. raw cashews
1¼ c. water
1 T. miso
2 T. lemon juice
2 T. tahini
¼ c. diced onion
1 t. garlic

½ t. salt
¼ c. nutritional yeast
2 T. olive or safflower oil
1 (12-oz.) package fettuccine, cooked
¼ c. vegan Parmesan cheese

1. Blend together cashews and water until completely smooth and creamy, about 90 seconds.
2. Add remaining ingredients, except oil, fettuccine noodles, and vegan Parmesan cheese. Purée until smooth. Slowly add oil until thick and oil is emulsified.
3. Heat in a saucepan over low heat for 4–5 minutes, stirring frequently. Serve over cooked fettuccine noodles and top with vegan Parmesan cheese.

PER SERVING Calories **558** Fat **20G** Protein **17G** Sodium **1,107MG** Fiber **5G** Carbohydrates **76G** Sugar **3G** Zinc **3MG** Calcium **40MG** Iron **4MG** Vit. D **0MCG** Vit. B$_{12}$ **0MCG**

VEGAN CHEESE SAUCES

Most vegan alfredo recipes start with a roux of margarine and soy milk, but this one uses cashew cream instead for a sensually decadent white sauce. The nutritional yeast is what adds the satisfying cheesy flavor in this recipe, so use it generously! Go ahead and lick the spoons; nobody's watching. Make a double batch of the sauce tonight to use in tomorrow night's gourmet lasagna.

What I Ate

DATE [　　] | [　　] | [　　]

TIME	FOOD ITEM	AMOUNT	CALORIES	FAT	CARBS	FIBER	PROTEIN
		TOTAL					

Today's Vegan Plate

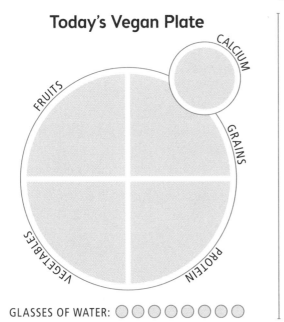

CALCIUM

FRUITS

GRAINS

VEGETABLES

PROTEIN

Thoughts about Today

GLASSES OF WATER: ○○○○○○○○

MENU

BREAKFAST	LUNCH	SNACK	DINNER
2 slices **Fat-Free Banana Bread**, 1 c. cashew milk	Hummus wrap with ½ c. spinach, ¼ c. tomatoes, 1 avocado sliced, 1 oz. olives, and ½ c. sprouts in a large flour tortilla; 3 oz. baby carrots	3 oz. **Spicy Roasted Chickpeas**	8 oz. **White Spinach Lasagna**, 1 c. steamed broccoli with 16g nutritional yeast, 1 c. orange juice

FAT-FREE BANANA BREAD

Yields 1 loaf

Add in ½ cup of walnuts or chocolate chips before baking for extra yumminess.

4 medium bananas, ripe	2 c. all-purpose flour
1/3 c. unsweetened soy milk	1 t. baking powder
	½ t. baking soda
2/3 c. sugar	½ t. salt
1 t. vanilla	¾ t. cinnamon

1. Preheat oven to 350°F. Lightly grease a loaf pan.
2. Mix together bananas, soy milk, sugar, and vanilla until smooth and creamy.
3. In a separate bowl, combine flour, baking powder, baking soda, and salt.
4. Combine the flour and banana mixtures.
5. Spread batter in loaf pan and sprinkle the top with cinnamon. Bake for about 55 minutes.

PER SERVING (1 SLICE) Calories **112** Fat **0G** Protein **2G** Sodium **130MG** Fiber **1G** Carbohydrates **26G** Sugar **12G** Zinc **0MG** Calcium **26MG** Iron **1MG** Vit. D **0MCG** Vit. B$_{12}$ **0MCG**

SPICY ROASTED CHICKPEAS

Serves 5

This unique take on chickpeas is easily customizable if you prefer other spices.

1 (14-oz.) can chickpeas, drained and rinsed	½ t. chili powder
	¼ t. salt
2 t. olive oil	¼ t. cayenne pepper

1. Preheat oven to 350°F. Toss chickpeas with olive oil. Add remaining ingredients and toss again.
2. Transfer chickpeas to a baking sheet and bake in the oven for 35–40 minutes, or until crunchy.

PER SERVING Calories **85** Fat **3G** Protein **4G** Sodium **228MG** Fiber **3G** Carbohydrates **11G** Sugar **2G** Zinc **0MG** Calcium **22MG** Iron : **1MG** Vit. D : **0MCG** Vit. B$_{12}$ **0MCG**

WHITE SPINACH LASAGNA

Serves 4

The spinach and cashews make this even more nutritious than the traditional version.

½ medium onion, diced	2 c. unsweetened soy milk
4 cloves garlic, minced	
2 T. olive oil	1 T. miso
1 (10-oz.) box frozen spinach, thawed and pressed	2 T. soy sauce
	2 T. lemon juice
½ t. salt	3 T. nutritional yeast
1 (14-oz.) block firm tofu, crumbled	2 t. onion powder
	1 (12-oz.) package lasagna noodles
¾ c. cashew butter	

1. Sauté onion and garlic in olive oil until soft. Add spinach, salt, and tofu and heat through. Cool completely.
2. In a small saucepan over low heat, combine remaining ingredients except for noodles until smooth and creamy.
3. Prepare lasagna noodles according to package instructions, and preheat oven to 350°F.
4. In a greased lasagna pan, layer cashew sauce, noodles, and spinach repeatedly. Top layer should be spinach then sauce.
5. Bake for 40 minutes. Allow to cool for at least 10 minutes before serving to allow lasagna to set.

PER SERVING Calories **861** Fat **41G** Protein **36G** Sodium **1,410MG** Fiber **10G** Carbohydrates **92G** Sugar **8G** Zinc **5 MG** Calcium **429 MG** Iron **9 MG** Vit. D **0MCG** Vit. B$_{12}$ **5MCG**

What I Ate

DATE ____ | ____ | ____

TIME	FOOD ITEM	AMOUNT	CALORIES	FAT	CARBS	FIBER	PROTEIN
TOTAL							

Today's Vegan Plate

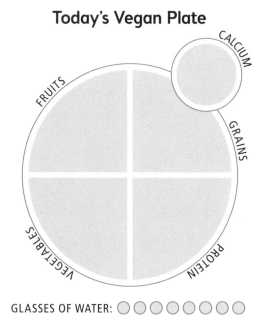

Thoughts about Today

GLASSES OF WATER: ○○○○○○○○

REVIEW

I FEEL:

_____

_____

_____

_____

MY GREATEST FOOD DISCOVERY THIS WEEK WAS:

_____

_____

_____

_____

THIS WEEK'S BIGGEST VEGAN CHALLENGE WAS:

_____

_____

_____

_____

NEW FOOD I'D LIKE TO TRY:

_____

_____

_____

_____

WHEN I LOOK BACK AT THIS WEEK, I MOST WANT TO REMEMBER:

_____

_____

_____

_____

HOW ARE YOU PROGRESSING TOWARD YOUR GOALS?

_____

_____

_____

_____

WEEK 7

You've learned quite a bit about preparing nutritious whole foods, have been eating a wide variety of fruits, vegetables, and healthy whole grains, and any cravings you have are beginning to subside. If not, you know plenty about meat and dairy substitutes and know how to satisfy a craving without giving up your fabulous new vegan diet.

Now that you've had plenty of time to ease into eating vegan, try adapting things a bit more to your personal tastes. Notice what works best for you, and begin listening to your own body and venturing out a bit more in the grocery store aisles. Try a few more store-bought substitutes, and, just for fun, see if you can find a vegetable or two you still haven't tried.

You know by now what foods are vegan, and which aren't, and you're used to eating well-balanced meals. Now that you're settled into your vegan ways, you're not likely to slip up, but for extra motivation, now's the time to buy a new vegan cookbook to get inspired, subscribe to a few new e-newsletters, or just spend some extra time browsing vegan groups on *Facebook* or find other like-minded people on *Instagram*.

Let's keep a good thing going this week! You've made it this far—you can make it for life!

MENU

BREAKFAST	LUNCH	SNACK	DINNER
1 slice **Fat-Free Banana Bread** (see recipe in Week 6, Sun.), 1 apple, 1 c. orange juice	8 oz. leftover **White Spinach Lasagna** (see recipe in Week 6, Sun.), 1 small baked potato with 16g nutritional yeast	Mixed vegetables (½ cucumber, 2 oz. baby carrots, ½ c. broccoli) with 2 T. hummus	1 c. **Pineapple Glazed Tofu**, 1 c. rice noodles

PINEAPPLE GLAZED TOFU

Serves 3

If you like orange chicken or sweet-and-sour dishes, try this saucy-sweet Pineapple Glazed Tofu, which is also excellent for kids. Toss with some noodles, rice, or add some diced vegetables to make it an entrée.

½ c. pineapple preserves
2 T. balsamic vinegar
2 T. soy sauce
⅔ c. pineapple juice

1 (14-oz.) block firm or extra-firm tofu, cubed
3 T. all-purpose flour
2 T. olive oil
1 t. cornstarch

1. Whisk together pineapple preserves, vinegar, soy sauce, and pineapple juice.
2. Coat tofu in flour, then sauté in olive oil for a few minutes, just until lightly golden. Reduce heat to medium low and add pineapple sauce, stirring well to combine and coat tofu.
3. Heat for 3–4 minutes, stirring frequently, then add cornstarch, whisking to combine and avoid lumps. Heat for a few more minutes, stirring until sauce has thickened.

PER SERVING Calories **419** Fat **16G** Protein **15G** Sodium **595MG** Fiber **2G** Carbohydrates **54G** Sugar **40G** Zinc **0MG** Calcium **117MG** Iron **3MG** Vit. D **0MCG** Vit. B$_{12}$ **0MCG**

RAISING HEALTHY VEGAN KIDS

Similar to adults, vegan children have several health advantages when eating a plant-based diet. Even the American Dietetic Association agrees: "Well-planned vegan and other types of vegetarian diets are appropriate for all stages of the life cycle, including during pregnancy, lactation, infancy, childhood, and adolescence." Kids are naturally compassionate, and on a healthy vegan diet, kids have a reduced risk for heart disease, cancer, obesity, diabetes. For vegan children's literature, check out *That's Why We Don't Eat Animals* by Ruby Roth, and *Vegan Lunch Box* by Jennifer McCann.

What I Ate

DATE [   ] | [   ] | [   ]

TIME	FOOD ITEM	AMOUNT	CALORIES	FAT	CARBS	FIBER	PROTEIN
	TOTAL						

Today's Vegan Plate

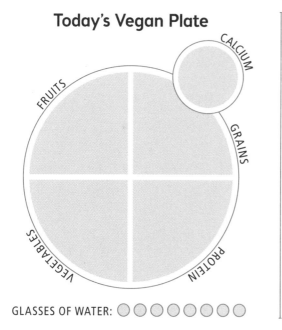

GLASSES OF WATER: ○○○○○○○○○

Thoughts about Today

MENU

BREAKFAST	LUNCH	SNACK	DINNER
1 c. instant Cream of Wheat with 1 banana, 1 c. soy hot chocolate	1¾ c. **Greek Salad with Vegan Feta Cheese** (see recipe in Week 2, Mon.) with 1 c. romaine lettuce; 1 c. pineapple; 1 c. unsweetened applesauce	1 slice **Fat-Free Banana Bread** (see recipe in Week 6, Sun.), 1 oz. cashews	6 oz. **Massaman Curried Seitan**, 1 c. brown rice

MASSAMAN CURRIED SEITAN

Serves 6

With Indian influences and popular among Muslim communities in Southern Thailand, massaman curry is a truly global dish. This version is simplified, but it still has a distinct kick. Diced tomatoes, broccoli, baby corn, or green peas would go well in this recipe if you want to add vegetables. Serve atop rice.

1 T. Chinese five-spice powder	2 medium sweet potatoes, chopped
½ t. fresh ginger, grated	1½ c. seitan, chopped small
½ t. turmeric	¼ t. cinnamon
¼ t. cayenne pepper, or to taste	2 whole cloves
1 T. olive oil	1 t. salt
1½ c. regular coconut milk, unsweetened	1 T. peanut butter
1 c. vegetable broth	2 t. brown sugar
	⅓ c. cashews

1. In a large skillet or stockpot, heat five-spice powder, ginger, turmeric, and cayenne pepper in olive oil for just 1 minute, stirring constantly until fragrant.
2. Reduce heat to medium low and add coconut milk and vegetable broth, stirring to combine. Add potatoes, seitan, cinnamon, cloves, and salt. Cover, and cook for 15–20 minutes, stirring occasionally.
3. Uncover, add peanut butter, sugar, and cashews, and heat for 1 more minute.
4. If you prefer a thicker curry, dissolve 1 T. cornstarch in 3 T. water and add to curry, simmering for 2–3 minutes until thick.

PER SERVING Calories **205** Fat **8G** Protein **14G** Sodium **712MG** Fiber **3G** Carbohydrates **20G** Sugar **5G** Zinc **1MG** Calcium **76MG** Iron **2MG** Vit. D **1MCG** Vit. B$_{12}$ **1MCG**

NO MORE BORING GREEN SALADS

Stock up on vegan salad dressings (or make a few of your own) so you'll always be ready. Try a Mexican-themed green salad with crumbled tortilla chips, salsa, and avocado. Add corn kernels and black beans for a Tex-Mex feel, and season with chili powder. Go Greek with olives, red onions, fresh oregano, and artichoke hearts. Try a sweet treat salad with diced apples or tangerine slices, candied walnuts, and dried cranberries.

What I Ate

DATE

TIME	FOOD ITEM	AMOUNT	CALORIES	FAT	CARBS	FIBER	PROTEIN
	TOTAL						

Today's Vegan Plate

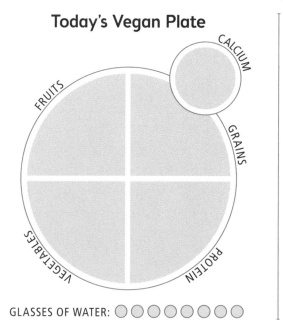

CALCIUM

FRUITS

GRAINS

VEGETABLES

PROTEIN

GLASSES OF WATER: ○○○○○○○○○

Thoughts about Today

MENU

BREAKFAST	LUNCH	SNACK	DINNER
1 English muffin with 1 vegan sausage patty, 1 (1-oz.) slice vegan cheese, 1 c. oat milk	Rice salad with 1 c. leftover brown rice, 1 c. mixed vegetables (½ cucumber, 2 oz. baby carrots, ½ c. broccoli), and 2 T. Goddess Dressing (see recipe in Week 1, Mon.); 1 c. strawberries; 1 c. tomato juice (no salt added)	1 pita with 2 T. hummus	¼ recipe Creamed Spinach and Mushrooms, 1 c. quinoa, 1 slice whole grain bread, toasted

CREAMED SPINACH AND MUSHROOMS

Serves 4

The combination of greens and nutritional yeast is simply delicious and provides an excellent jolt of nutrients that vegans need. Don't forget that spinach will shrink when cooked, so use lots!

½ medium onion, diced
2 cloves garlic, minced
1½ c. sliced white button mushrooms
2 T. olive oil
1 T. all-purpose flour
2 bunches fresh spinach, trimmed

1 c. unsweetened soy milk
1 T. vegan margarine
¼ t. nutmeg
2 T. nutritional yeast
1 t. salt
1 t. black pepper

1. Sauté onion, garlic, and mushrooms in olive oil for 3–4 minutes. Add flour and heat, stirring constantly, for 1 minute.
2. Reduce heat to medium low and add spinach and soy milk. Cook uncovered for 8–10 minutes until spinach is soft and liquid has reduced.
3. Stir in margarine, nutmeg, and nutritional yeast, and season with salt and pepper.

PER SERVING Calories **163** Fat **11G** Protein **8G** Sodium **730MG** Fiber **4G** Carbohydrates **11G** Sugar **2G** Zinc **2MG** Calcium **261MG** Iron **5MG** Vit. D **.0MCG** Vit. B_{12} **3MCG**

BORED OF HUMMUS?

Spice up hummus by stirring in a few minced roasted red peppers, marinated garlic, sun-dried tomatoes, Indian seasonings, minced chipotles or jalapeños, or a sprinkle of fresh herbs—just about any kind will do.

What I Ate

DATE [ ] | [ ] | [ ]

TIME	FOOD ITEM	AMOUNT	CALORIES	FAT	CARBS	FIBER	PROTEIN
	TOTAL						

Today's Vegan Plate

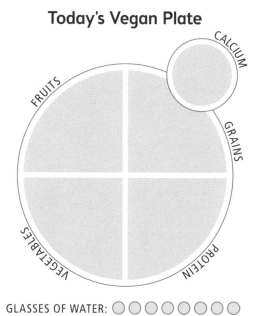

Thoughts about Today

GLASSES OF WATER: ○ ○ ○ ○ ○ ○ ○ ○

MENU

BREAKFAST	LUNCH	SNACK	DINNER
1½ c. **Tropical Breakfast Couscous** (see recipe in Week 2, Fri.), 1 banana, 1 c. soy milk	Sandwich with 1 oz. **Sun-Dried Tomato Pesto** (see recipe in Week 2, Mon.), 1 oz. avocado, ¼ tomato, 1 slice purple onion, 4 slices of cucumber, and 1 c. sprouts on 2 slices whole grain bread	1 oz. dried apricots, 2 oz. cashews	1½ c. **White Bean and Orzo Minestrone Soup**

WHITE BEAN AND ORZO MINESTRONE SOUP

Serves 6

Italian minestrone is a simple and universally loved soup. This version uses tiny orzo pasta, cannellini beans, and plenty of vegetables.

3 cloves garlic, minced
1 medium onion, chopped
2 stalks celery, chopped
2 T. olive oil
5 c. vegetable broth
1 medium carrot, diced
1 c. green beans, chopped
2 small red potatoes, chopped small

2 medium tomatoes, chopped
1 (15-oz.) can cannellini beans, drained
1 t. dried basil
½ t. dried oregano
¾ c. orzo
1 t. salt
1 t. black pepper

1. In a large soup pot, heat garlic, onion, and celery in olive oil until just soft, about 3–4 minutes.
2. Add vegetable broth, carrot, green beans, potatoes, tomatoes, beans, basil, and oregano, and bring to a simmer. Cover, and cook on medium-low heat for 20–25 minutes.
3. Add orzo and heat another 10 minutes, just until orzo is cooked. Season with salt and pepper.

PER SERVING Calories **223** Fat **6G** Protein **8G** Sodium **1,053MG** Fiber **5G** Carbohydrates **36G** Sugar **7G** Zinc **1MG** Calcium **60MG** Iron **2MG** Vit. D **0MCG** Vit. B$_{12}$ **0MCG**

SANDWICH SUBSTITUTES

Vegan deli meat slices are available everywhere— from your local grocery store to retailers such as Target and Walmart. Lightlife, Tofurky, and Yves all make delicious plant-based deli slices.

What I Ate

DATE ▢ | ▢ | ▢

TIME	FOOD ITEM	AMOUNT	CALORIES	FAT	CARBS	FIBER	PROTEIN
	TOTAL						

Today's Vegan Plate

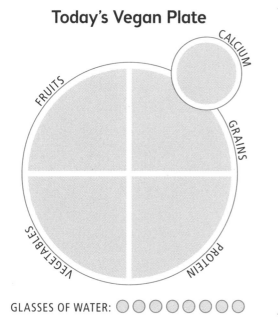

GLASSES OF WATER: ◯◯◯◯◯◯◯◯

Thoughts about Today

BREAKFAST	LUNCH	SNACK	DINNER
1 avocado, mashed, on 2 slices of whole grain toast with 1 t. sea salt sprinkled on top; 1 apple or 1 banana	1½ c. leftover White Bean and Orzo Minestrone Soup (see recipe in Week 7, Thurs.)	1 c. yogurt with ⅓ c. granola, 1 oz. almonds	6 oz. Easy Pad Thai Noodles

EASY PAD THAI NOODLES

Serves 6

Volumes could be written about Thailand's national dish. It's sweet, sour, spicy, and salty all at once, and filled with as much texture and flavor as the streets of Bangkok themselves. Try topping this with bean sprouts, crushed toasted peanuts, extra scallions, or sliced lime.

1 lb. thin rice noodles
Hot water for soaking
¼ c. tahini
¼ c. ketchup
¼ c. soy sauce
2 T. white vinegar
3 T. lime juice
2 T. sugar

¾ t. crushed red pepper flakes
1 (14-oz.) block firm or extra-firm tofu, diced small
3 cloves garlic, minced
¼ c. vegetable oil
4 scallions, chopped
½ t. salt

1. Cover noodles in hot water and set aside to soak until soft, about 5 minutes.
2. Whisk together tahini, ketchup, soy sauce, vinegar, lime juice, sugar, and red pepper flakes.
3. In a large skillet, fry tofu and garlic in oil until tofu is lightly golden brown. Add noodles, stirring to combine well, and fry for 2–3 minutes.
4. Reduce heat to medium and add tahini and ketchup sauce mixture, stirring well to combine. Allow to cook for 3–4 minutes until well combined and heated through. Add scallions and salt. Heat 1 more minute, stirring well, before serving.

PER SERVING Calories **516** Fat **19G** Protein **14G** Sodium **921MG** Fiber **3G** Carbohydrates **74G** Sugar **8G** Zinc **1MG** Calcium **89MG** Iron **2MG** Vit. D **0MCG** Vit. B$_{12}$ **0MCG**

KNOW YOUR NOODLES

Rice noodles cook quicker than pasta, so they're great when you're superhungry or in a hurry. Many grocery stores, as well as Asian markets stock shirataki noodles—a high-protein, low-carb thin, translucent noodle made from tofu that doesn't need to be cooked—perfect for hungry vegans to slurp! Check the refrigerator section for these.

What I Ate

DATE [ ] | [ ] | [ ]

TIME	FOOD ITEM	AMOUNT	CALORIES	FAT	CARBS	FIBER	PROTEIN
		TOTAL					

Today's Vegan Plate

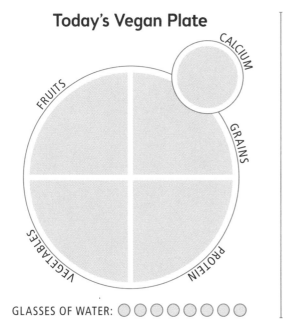

CALCIUM

FRUITS

GRAINS

VEGETABLES

PROTEIN

GLASSES OF WATER: ○○○○○○○○

Thoughts about Today

MENU

BREAKFAST	LUNCH	SNACK	DINNER
6 oz. **Baked "Sausage" and Mushroom Frittata**, 1 banana	6 oz. leftover **Easy Pad Thai Noodles** (see recipe in Week 7, Fri.)	1 c. edamame, 2 oz. dried cranberries	5 oz. **Super-Quick Black Bean Soup**, 1 c. roasted butternut squash

BAKED "SAUSAGE" AND MUSHROOM FRITTATA

Serves 6

Baked tofu frittatas are an easy brunch or weekend breakfast. Once you've got the technique down, it's easy to adjust the ingredients to your liking. With tofu and mock meat, this one packs a super protein punch!

½ medium yellow onion, diced

3 cloves garlic, minced

½ c. sliced white button mushrooms

1 (12-oz.) package vegan sausage substitute

2 T. olive oil

¾ t. salt

¼ t. black pepper

1 (14-oz.) block firm or extra-firm tofu

1 (14-oz.) block silken tofu

1 T. soy sauce

2 T. nutritional yeast

¼ t. turmeric

1 medium tomato, sliced thin

1. Preheat oven to 325°F and lightly grease a glass pie pan.
2. Heat onion, garlic, mushrooms, and vegan sausage in olive oil in a large skillet for 3–4 minutes until sausage is browned and mushrooms are soft. Season with salt and pepper and set aside.
3. Combine firm tofu, silken tofu, soy sauce, nutritional yeast, and turmeric in a blender, and process until mixed. Combine tofu with sausage mixture and spread into pan. Layer slices of tomato on top.
4. Bake in oven for about 45 minutes, or until firm. Allow to cool for 5–10 minutes before serving, as frittata will set as it cools.

PER SERVING Calories **485** Fat **21G** Protein **32G** Sodium **1,385MG** Fiber **10G** Carbohydrates **42G** Sugar **1G** Zinc **0MG** Calcium **252MG** Iron **7MG** Vit. D **0MCG** Vit. B$_{12}$ **1MCG**

SUPER-QUICK BLACK BEAN SOUP

Serves 6

When you want a hot meal quickly, try this rich and thick soup.

2 (15-oz.) cans black beans, undrained

1 c. vegetable broth

⅔ c. salsa

½ t. garlic powder

1 T. chili powder

¼ t. salt

1 T. chopped fresh cilantro

1. Using a potato masher or a large fork, coarsely mash 1 can of beans.
2. In a medium saucepan, combine the mashed beans with the remaining whole beans, vegetable broth, salsa, garlic powder, chili powder, and salt. Simmer for 10 minutes, just until well combined and heated through. Serve topped with fresh chopped cilantro.

PER SERVING Calories **143** Fat **1G** Protein **9G** Sodium **991MG** Fiber **11G** Carbohydrates **26G** Sugar **2G** Zinc **1MG** Calcium **64MG** Iron **3MG** Vit. D **0MCG** Vit. B$_{12}$ **0MCG**

What I Ate

DATE ____ | ____ | ____

TIME	FOOD ITEM	AMOUNT	CALORIES	FAT	CARBS	FIBER	PROTEIN
	TOTAL						

Today's Vegan Plate

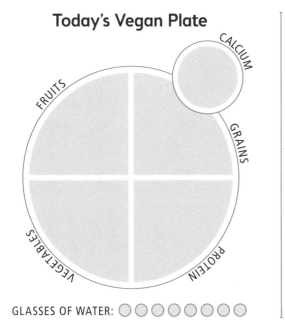

GLASSES OF WATER: ○○○○○○○○

Thoughts about Today

MENU

BREAKFAST	LUNCH	SNACK	DINNER
1 Blueberry Muffin; mixed fruit salad with ¼ c. grapes, ½ tangerine, ½ diced apple, ½ banana, ¼ c. chopped cantaloupe; 1 c. hemp milk	5 oz. leftover Super-Quick Black Bean Soup (see recipe in Week 7, Sat.); ½ lb. collard greens sautéed with ½ T. coconut oil, 1 clove minced garlic, and 16g nutritional yeast; 1 slice whole grain toast	9 oz. Fresh Basil Bruschetta	10 oz. Sweet-and-Sour Tempeh, ½ c. brown rice or quinoa

BLUEBERRY MUFFINS

Yields 1½ dozen muffins

These moist muffins will become a favorite!

2 c. whole wheat flour
1 c. all-purpose flour
1¼ c. sugar
1 T. baking powder
1 t. salt

1½ c. unsweetened soy milk
½ c. unsweetened applesauce
½ t. vanilla
2 c. blueberries, divided

1. Preheat oven to 400°F. In a large bowl, combine flours, sugar, baking powder, and salt. Set aside.
2. Combine wet ingredients, and whisk until mixed.
3. Combine wet and dry ingredients. Fold in 1 c. berries.
4. Divide batter into lined muffin tins; top with 1 c. berries. Bake for 20–25 minutes, or until lightly golden.

PER SERVING (1 MUFFIN) Calories 144 Fat 1G Protein 3G Sodium 198MG Fiber 2G Carbohydrates 33G Sugar 16G Zinc 0MG Calcium 88MG Iron 1MG Vit. D 0MCG Vit. B$_{12}$ 0MCG

FRESH BASIL BRUSCHETTA

Serves 4

Try this as an appetizer on a warm day.

¾ c. balsamic vinegar
1 T. sugar
2 large tomatoes, diced
3 cloves garlic, minced
2 T. olive oil

¼ c. chopped fresh basil
1 t. salt
1 t. black pepper
10 slices French bread

1. Whisk vinegar and sugar in saucepan. Boil, then simmer for 6–8 minutes. Remove from heat.
2. Combine tomatoes, garlic, olive oil, basil, salt, and pepper in bowl. Gently toss with balsamic sauce.
3. Spoon tomato and balsamic mixture over bread.

PER SERVING Calories 570 Fat 11G Protein 18G Sodium 1,561MG Fiber 5G Carbohydrates 99G Sugar 20G Zinc 2MG Calcium 112MG Iron 7MG Vit. D 0MCG Vit. B$_{12}$ 0MCG

SWEET-AND-SOUR TEMPEH

Serves 4

Serve over rice, if desired.

1 c. vegetable broth
2 T. soy sauce
1 (8-oz.) package tempeh
2 T. barbecue sauce
½ t. ground ginger
2 T. maple syrup
⅓ c. rice vinegar
1 T. cornstarch

1 (15-oz.) can pineapple chunks, juice reserved
2 T. olive oil
1 medium green bell pepper, chopped
1 medium red bell pepper, chopped
1 medium yellow onion, chopped

1. Whisk broth and soy sauce. Bring to simmer in large skillet. Add tempeh and simmer for 10 minutes. Remove tempeh from pan. Reserve ½ c. broth mix.
2. In a small bowl, whisk barbecue sauce, ginger, maple syrup, vinegar, cornstarch, and juice from pineapples until cornstarch is dissolved. Set aside.
3. Heat oil, tempeh, peppers, and onion in skillet. Sauté for 1 minute. Add sauce and bring to simmer.
4. Allow to cook until sauce thickens, about 6–8 minutes. Reduce heat and stir in pineapples.

PER SERVING Calories 317 Fat 13G Protein 14G Sodium 701MG Fiber 3G Carbohydrates 40G Sugar 28G Zinc 1MG Calcium 106MG Iron 2MG Vit. D 0MCG Vit. B$_{12}$ 0MCG

What I Ate

DATE [ ] | [ ] | [ ]

TIME	FOOD ITEM	AMOUNT	CALORIES	FAT	CARBS	FIBER	PROTEIN
		TOTAL					

Today's Vegan Plate

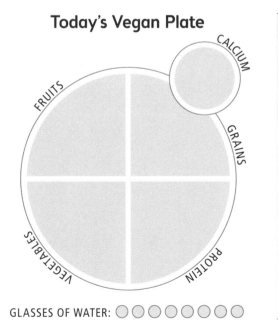

CALCIUM

FRUITS

GRAINS

VEGETABLES

PROTEIN

GLASSES OF WATER: ○○○○○○○○

Thoughts about Today

I FEEL:

_____

_____

_____

_____

MY GREATEST FOOD DISCOVERY THIS WEEK WAS:

_____

_____

_____

_____

THIS WEEK'S BIGGEST VEGAN CHALLENGE WAS:

_____

_____

_____

_____

NEW FOOD I'D LIKE TO TRY:

_____

_____

_____

_____

WHEN I LOOK BACK AT THIS WEEK, I MOST WANT TO REMEMBER:

_____

_____

_____

_____

HOW ARE YOU PROGRESSING TOWARD YOUR GOALS?

_____

_____

_____

_____

WEEK 8

You've been vegan almost two months now. Can you believe it? You're two-thirds of the way through this planner and hopefully well on the way to achieving your goals. How does it feel? Sometimes, our daily lives are so hectic and busy that we barely have a moment to stop and relax, much less to really take time out to think. This week, set aside an hour or two to take a self-care break. Find a quiet spot or go for a meditative walk, whether it's at a city park, the beach, or a mountain trail. Turn off your cell phone and just be. Let your mind process the journey that you've undertaken, and appreciate just how far you've come and changed as a person. Reflect on how your experiences over the past eight weeks have changed you, and what you hope to achieve over the next few weeks to come. Do you feel content as a vegan? Was it easier or harder than you thought? Has it been worth it so far? Is it more or less fulfilling than you thought it would be? What will be the next step for you?

If this isn't something you normally do, you'll be surprised just how nourishing a couple of hours of fresh air, nature, and mental solitude can be. Don't forget to pack a healthy snack!

MENU

BREAKFAST	LUNCH	SNACK	DINNER
2 **Blueberry Muffins** (see recipe in Week 7, Sun.), 1 banana, 1 c. soy milk	1 c. store-bought vegan chili (approximately 250 calories), 1 c. steamed broccoli with 16g nutritional yeast	Mixed vegetables (½ cucumber, 2 oz. baby carrots, ½ c. broccoli) with 2 T. hummus	1 c. **Vietnamese Noodle Salad**, 1 c. steamed spinach, 1 c. orange juice

VIETNAMESE NOODLE SALAD

Serves 2

This light but filling salad has a bit of heat from the red pepper flakes—add more if you like it even hotter!

- **12 Beyond Chicken grilled chicken strips**
- **4 oz. bean thread noodles, softened in hot water for 20 minutes**
- **½ c. thinly sliced scallions**
- **½ c. fresh cilantro**
- **1 T. crushed red pepper flakes**
- **2 T. lime juice**
- **2 T. soy sauce**
- **1 T. pickled garlic, chopped**
- **Sugar to taste**

1. Grill vegan chicken strips for a few minutes on each side (or according to package instructions) until well marked, then chop into thin strips.
2. Drain the soaked and softened noodles. Combine the noodles, chicken strips, scallions, cilantro, and crushed red pepper into a serving bowl.
3. Mix together the lime juice, soy sauce, pickled garlic, and sugar, and toss with the salad ingredients.

PER SERVING Calories **364** Fat **4G** Protein **22G** Sodium **1,220MG** Fiber **5G** Carbohydrates **60G** Sugar **1G** Zinc **1MG** Calcium **90MG** Iron **5MG** Vit. D **0MCG** Vit. B$_{12}$ **0MCG**

THE PERFECT GREEN

If you think spinach is too slimy and kale is too bitter, have you tried Swiss chard? Chard contains 18 milligrams of calcium, 25 mg of magnesium, and 298mcg of vitamin K (that's 3 times the recommended daily intake of vitamin K!). It's quicker cooking than collards, but with a milder flavor than kale or mustard greens. Try it steamed with a bit of garlic, olive oil, and lemon juice, or smothered in nutritional yeast or vegan Parmesan.

What I Ate

DATE [ ] | [ ] | [ ]

TIME	FOOD ITEM	AMOUNT	CALORIES	FAT	CARBS	FIBER	PROTEIN
	TOTAL						

Today's Vegan Plate

CALCIUM

FRUITS

GRAINS

VEGETABLES

PROTEIN

GLASSES OF WATER: ○○○○○○○○

Thoughts about Today

BREAKFAST	LUNCH	SNACK	DINNER
1 c. whole grain cereal with ½ c. cashew milk	½ c. **Tempeh Dill "Chicken" Salad** (see recipe in Week 5, Thurs.) on 2 slices whole grain bread with ¼ tomato, sliced, and ¼ c. iceberg lettuce; 10 pita chips	200 calories of pretzels; mixed fruit salad with ½ apple, ½ banana, ½ c. strawberries, and ½ c. pineapple	17 oz. **Spaghetti with Italian "Meatballs"**

SPAGHETTI WITH ITALIAN "MEATBALLS"

Serves 4

These little TVP nuggets are so chewy and addicting, you just might want to make a double batch. If you can't find beef-flavored bouillon, just use what you've got. Don't be tempted to add extra water to the TVP, as it needs to be a little dry for this recipe. If you are short on time, you can find vegan "meatballs" in the freezer section of your local grocery store (try Gardein's frozen Classic Meatless Meatballs).

½ vegan beef-flavored bouillon cube
⅔ c. hot water
⅔ c. TVP
4 T. unsweetened apple-sauce (for replacement of 2 eggs)
½ medium onion, minced
2 T. ketchup
½ t. garlic powder
1 t. dried basil
1 t. dried parsley
½ t. dried sage
½ t. salt
½ c. bread crumbs
¾ c. all-purpose flour
2 t. olive oil for panfrying
3 c. prepared spaghetti sauce
1 12 oz. package spaghetti noodles, cooked

1. Dissolve bouillon cube in hot water, and pour over TVP to reconstitute. Allow to sit for 6–7 minutes. Gently press to remove any excess moisture.
2. In a large bowl, combine TVP, applesauce, onion, ketchup sauce, and seasonings until well mixed.
3. Add bread crumbs and combine well, then add flour, a few tablespoons at a time, mixing well to combine until mixture is sticky and thick. You may need a little more or less than ½ cup.
4. Using lightly floured hands, shape into balls 1½"–2" thick.
5. Panfry "meatballs" in a bit of olive oil over medium heat, rolling them around in the pan to maintain the shape until golden brown on all sides.
6. Reduce heat to medium low and add spaghetti sauce, heating thoroughly. Serve over cooked spaghetti noodles.

PER SERVING Calories **613** Fat **8G** Protein **26G** Sodium **1,514MG** Fiber **11G** Carbohydrates **108G** Sugar **17G** Zinc **2MG** Calcium **131MG** Iron **7MG** Vit. D **0MCG** Vit. B₁₂ **0MCG**

HUMAN RIGHTS, ANIMAL RIGHTS

Many social-justice activists, including notable heroes Coretta Scott King, Angela Davis, Rosa Parks, and Cesar Chavez, all rejected animal exploitation as a logical extension of their belief in equality. In the words of Albert Einstein, they have "widened the circle of compassion" to include all victims of oppression and injustice—animals and humans alike.

What I Ate

DATE [   ] | [   ] | [   ]

TIME	FOOD ITEM	AMOUNT	CALORIES	FAT	CARBS	FIBER	PROTEIN
	TOTAL						

Today's Vegan Plate

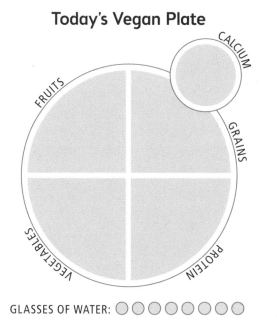

CALCIUM
FRUITS
GRAINS
PROTEIN
VEGETABLES

GLASSES OF WATER: ○○○○○○○○

Thoughts about Today

MENU

BREAKFAST	LUNCH	SNACK	DINNER
2 T. vegan cream cheese, 1 T. sugar-free jam on 2 slices whole grain toast, 1 c. tomato juice (no salt added)	1 baked potato with ½ c. black beans, ¼ c. salsa or guacamole, and 1 oz. vegan cheese; 1 c. orange juice	200 calories of whole grain crackers with 2 T. almond butter	6¼ oz. **Indian Tofu Palak** with ½ c. quinoa and 16g nutritional yeast

INDIAN TOFU PALAK

Serves 4

Palak paneer is a popular Indian dish of creamed spinach and soft cheese. This version uses tofu for a similar dish. Serve over basmati rice and with Indian flat bread, if desired.

3 cloves garlic, minced	2 (8-oz.) bags fresh
1 (14-oz.) block extra firm tofu, cut into small cubes	spinach
	3 T. water
	1 T. curry powder
2 T. olive oil	2 t. cumin
2 T. nutritional yeast	½ t. salt
1 t. garlic powder	½ c. plain soy yogurt
½ t. onion powder	

1. Heat garlic and tofu in olive oil over low heat and add nutritional yeast, garlic powder and onion powder, stirring to coat tofu. Heat for 2–3 minutes until tofu is lightly browned.
2. Add spinach, water, curry powder, cumin, and salt, stirring well to combine. Once spinach starts to wilt, add soy yogurt and heat just until spinach is fully wilted and soft.

PER SERVING Calories **242** Fat **13G** Protein **19G** Sodium **487MG** Fiber **9G** Carbohydrates **18G** Sugar **3G** Zinc **2MG** Calcium **538MG** Iron **12MG** Vit. D **0MCG** Vit. B$_{12}$ **2MCG**

INDIAN VEGAN OPTIONS

In India, many vegetarians forgo eggs as well as onions and garlic for religious purposes, making Indian food an excellent choice for vegans. When eating at Indian restaurants, be sure to ask about *ghee*, which is clarified butter, a traditional ingredient, but easily and frequently substituted with oil. You'll also want to be on the lookout for any yogurt or cream in sauces. Many Indian dishes are vegan-friendly, but double-check with your server if you are unsure!

What I Ate

DATE [   ] | [   ] | [   ]

TIME	FOOD ITEM	AMOUNT	CALORIES	FAT	CARBS	FIBER	PROTEIN
		TOTAL					

Today's Vegan Plate

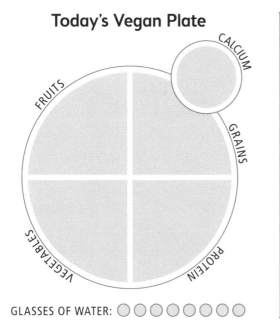

GLASSES OF WATER: ○○○○○○○○○

Thoughts about Today

BREAKFAST	LUNCH	SNACK	DINNER
½ c. oatmeal with 1 oz. almonds, 1 banana, 1 c. almond milk	6¼ oz. leftover Indian Tofu Palak (see recipe in Week 8, Wed.) with ½ c. quinoa	1 c. unsweetened applesauce, 1 oz. raisins	6 oz. Sweet and Spicy Peanut Noodles, 1 c. steamed broccoli

SWEET AND SPICY PEANUT NOODLES

Serves 4

Like the call of the siren, these noodles entice you with their sweet pineapple flavor, then scorch your tongue with fiery chilies. Very sneaky, indeed.

1 (12-oz.) package Asian-style noodles	1 t. fresh ginger, grated
⅓ c. peanut butter	½ t. salt
2 T. soy sauce	1 T. olive oil
⅔ c. pineapple juice	1 t. sesame oil
2 cloves garlic, minced	3 small chilies, minced
1 T. brown sugar	¾ c. diced pineapple

1. Prepare noodles according to package instructions and set aside.
2. In a small saucepan, stir together peanut butter, soy sauce, pineapple juice, garlic, brown sugar, ginger, and salt over low heat, just until well combined.
3. Place olive oil and sesame oil in a large skillet and fry minced chilies and pineapple for 2–3 minutes, stirring frequently until pineapple is lightly browned. Add noodles and fry for another minute, stirring well.
4. Reduce heat to low and add peanut butter sauce mixture, stirring to combine well. Heat for 1 more minute until well combined.

PER SERVING Calories **524** Fat **17G** Protein **11G** Sodium **770MG** Fiber **4G** Carbohydrates **86G** Sugar **13G** Zinc **1MG** Calcium **28MG** Iron **1MG** Vit. D **0MCG** Vit. B$_{12}$ **0MCG**

STAY MOTIVATED, STAY INFORMED

Bored and online? Take a few minutes to learn something new without cracking a book. *YouTube* is full of vegan cooking demonstrations, lectures, interviews, and plenty of pure comedic gold. Just type the word *vegan* into *YouTube*, and you'll be entertained for hours. Check out *Eco-Vegan Gal*, *Earthling Ed*, *Bite Size Vegan*, *Sweet Simple Vegan*, and *James Aspey's YouTube* channels to get started.

What I Ate

DATE [   ] | [   ] | [   ]

TIME	FOOD ITEM	AMOUNT	CALORIES	FAT	CARBS	FIBER	PROTEIN
TOTAL							

Today's Vegan Plate

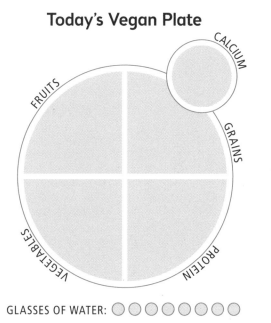

CALCIUM

FRUITS

GRAINS

VEGETABLES

PROTEIN

GLASSES OF WATER: ○ ○ ○ ○ ○ ○ ○ ○

Thoughts about Today

BREAKFAST	LUNCH	SNACK	DINNER
1 c. Cream of Wheat with 1 banana, 1 c. soy hot chocolate or orange juice	6 oz. leftover **Sweet and Spicy Peanut Noodles** (see recipe in Week 8, Thurs.), 1 c. pineapple	200 calories of whole grain chips with ½ c. salsa or guacamole	½ c. **Homemade Garlic and Herb Gnocchi** with 1 oz. **Sun-Dried Tomato Pesto** (see recipe in Week 2, Mon.); side green salad with 2 c. romaine lettuce, 1 tomato, 1 diced cucumber, and 2 T. **Goddess Dressing** (see recipe in Week 1, Mon.)

HOMEMADE GARLIC AND HERB GNOCCHI

Serves 4

Homemade gnocchi is well worth the effort if you have the time!

2 large russet potatoes	¾ t. salt
¾ t. garlic powder	1½ c. all-purpose flour
½ t. dried basil	Water for boiling
½ t. dried parsley	

1. Bake potatoes until done, about 50 minutes at 400°F. Allow to cool, then peel skins.
2. Using a fork, mash potatoes with garlic powder, basil, parsley, and salt until potatoes are completely smooth, with no lumps.
3. On a floured work surface, place half of the flour with the potatoes on top. Use your hands to work flour into the potatoes to form a dough. Only add as much flour as is needed to form a dough. Knead smooth.
4. Working in batches, roll out a rope of dough about 1" thick. Slice into 1"-long pieces, and gently roll against a fork to make grooves in the dough. This helps the sauce stick to the dough.
5. Cook gnocchi in boiling water for 2–3 minutes until they rise to the surface. Serve immediately.

PER SERVING Calories **319** Fat **1G** Protein **9G** Sodium **447MG** Fiber **4G** Carbohydrates **70G** Sugar **1G** Zinc **1MG** Calcium **33MG** Iron **4MG** Vit. D **0MCG** Vit. B_{12} **0MCG**

BAKED TORTILLA CHIPS

Instead of buying a bag of premade chips, grab a bag of whole wheat tortillas at the store, and make your own tortilla chips! Slice the tortillas into strips or triangles, and arrange in a single layer on a baking sheet. Drizzle with olive oil for a crispier chip, and season with a bit of salt and garlic powder if you want, or just bake them plain. It'll take about 5–6 minutes on each side in a 300°F oven.

What I Ate

DATE [   ] | [   ] | [   ]

TIME	FOOD ITEM	AMOUNT	CALORIES	FAT	CARBS	FIBER	PROTEIN
	TOTAL						

Today's Vegan Plate

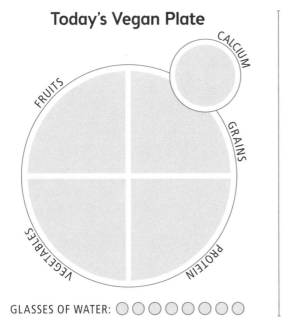

GLASSES OF WATER: ○○○○○○○○

Thoughts about Today

MENU

BREAKFAST	LUNCH	SNACK	DINNER
1 vegan sausage patty, 2 Quick and Easy Vegan Biscuits, 2 T. sugar-free jam	Vegan grilled cheese sandwich; side green salad with 2 c. romaine lettuce or other leafy green, 1 tomato, 1 diced cucumber, and 2 T. Goddess Dressing (see recipe in Week 1, Mon.)	1 pita, mixed vegetables (½ cucumber, 2 oz. baby carrots, ½ c. broccoli) with 2 T. hummus	Store-bought vegan chicken nuggets (about 450 calories), vegan mashed potatoes, 8 spears steamed asparagus

QUICK AND EASY VEGAN BISCUITS

Yields 14 biscuits

Use these multipurpose vegan biscuits to mop up your vegan gravy; or top with vegan margarine or jam, pour some Earl Grey, and enjoy a British afternoon tea.

2 c. all-purpose flour
3 t. baking powder
½ t. onion powder
½ t. garlic powder
½ t. salt
5 T. cold vegan margarine
⅔ c. unsweetened soy milk

1. Preheat oven to 425°F.
2. Combine flour, baking powder, onion powder, garlic powder, and salt in a large bowl. Add margarine.
3. Using a fork, mash margarine with the dry ingredients until crumbly.
4. Add soy milk a few tablespoons at a time and combine just until dough forms. You may need to add a little more or less than ⅔ cup.
5. Knead a few times on a floured surface, then roll out to ¾" thick. Cut into 3" rounds.
6. Bake for 12–14 minutes, or until done.

PER SERVING (1 BISCUIT) Calories 106 Fat 4G Protein 2G Sodium 208MG Fiber 1G Carbohydrates 14G Sugar 0G Zinc 0MG Calcium 90MG Iron 1MG Vit. D 0MCG Vit. B$_{12}$ 0MCG

IT'S GREAT TO BE VEGAN!

Most major cities have a summer vegan festival to celebrate all things vegan, which is typically referred to as a VegFest. VegFests are sure to be packed with lots of great food, vendors, speakers, fun, and lots of other vegans. Washington, DC, New York City, Los Angeles, Baltimore, and Atlanta all offer VegFests… and there are even international festivals such as in Australia, Belgium, the United Kingdom, France, and Germany! Find out when there's a vegan or Earth Day festival near you with a quick Google search, add it to your calendar and grab a friend to enjoy the day.

What I Ate

DATE [ ] | [ ] | [ ]

TIME	FOOD ITEM	AMOUNT	CALORIES	FAT	CARBS	FIBER	PROTEIN
	TOTAL						

Today's Vegan Plate

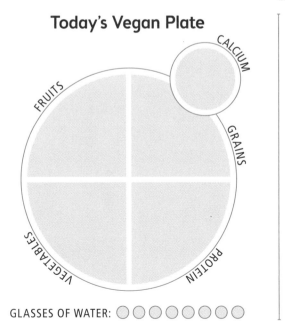

GLASSES OF WATER: ○○○○○○○○○

Thoughts about Today

BREAKFAST	LUNCH	SNACK	DINNER
1 c. whole grain cereal with ½ c. cashew milk	1 **Easy Vegan Pizza Bagels** (see recipe in Week 1, Wed.); Greek spinach salad with 2 c. fresh spinach, ½ red bell pepper, 2 T. black olives, ¼ c. chopped artichoke hearts, and 2 T. **Goddess Dressing** (see recipe in Week 1, Mon.)	2 leftover **Quick and Easy Vegan Biscuits** (see recipe in Week 8, Sat.), 2 T. sugar-free jam	1 c. **Chinese Fried Rice with Tofu and Cashews**, 1 c. pineapple

CHINESE FRIED RICE WITH TOFU AND CASHEWS

Serves 3

On busy weeknights, pick up some plain white rice from a Chinese takeout restaurant and turn it into a home-cooked meal in a jiffy. Garnish with fresh lime wedges and a sprinkle of sea salt and fresh black pepper on top.

2 cloves garlic, minced	3 T. soy sauce
1 (12-oz.) block silken tofu, cut into cubes	1 T. sesame oil
3 T. olive oil, divided	2 T. lime juice
3 c. leftover rice	3 scallions (greens and whites), sliced
½ c. frozen mixed diced vegetables	⅓ c. chopped cashews

1. In a large skillet or wok, sauté garlic and tofu in 2 tablespoons olive oil over medium high heat, stirring frequently until tofu is lightly browned, about 6–8 minutes.
2. Add remaining 1 tablespoon olive oil, rice, and vegetables, stirring well to combine.
3. Add soy sauce and sesame oil and combine well.
4. Allow to cook, stirring constantly, for 3–4 minutes.
5. Remove from heat and stir in remaining ingredients.

PER SERVING Calories **564** Fat **28G** Protein **14G** Sodium **888MG** Fiber **2G** Carbohydrates **64G** Sugar **3G** Zinc **2MG** Calcium **125MG** Iron **5MG** Vit. D **0MCG** Vit. B$_{12}$ **0MCG**

IS YOUR SOY CHEESE VEGAN?

Many nondairy products do actually contain dairy, even if it says "nondairy" right there on the package! Nondairy creamer and soy cheeses are notorious for this. Look for casein or whey (both proteins found in cow's milk) on the ingredients list, particularly if you suffer from dairy allergies, and, if you're allergic to soy, look for nut- or rice-based vegan cheeses, such as by Treeline Treenut Cheese or MozzaRisella. For other delicious plant-based cheese brands check out: Daiya, Miyoko's, Follow Your Heart, Kite-Hill, and Field Roast's Chao.

What I Ate

DATE [   ] | [   ] | [   ]

TIME	FOOD ITEM	AMOUNT	CALORIES	FAT	CARBS	FIBER	PROTEIN
TOTAL							

Today's Vegan Plate

Thoughts about Today

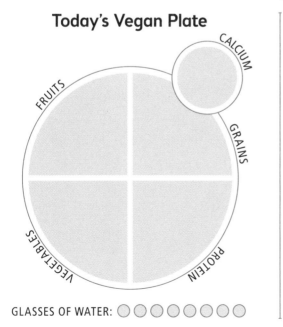

GLASSES OF WATER: ○○○○○○○○○

I FEEL:

MY GREATEST FOOD DISCOVERY THIS WEEK WAS:

THIS WEEK'S BIGGEST VEGAN CHALLENGE WAS:

NEW FOOD I'D LIKE TO TRY:

WHEN I LOOK BACK AT THIS WEEK, I MOST WANT TO REMEMBER:

HOW ARE YOU PROGRESSING TOWARD YOUR GOALS?

WEEK 9

You've come a long way, and you have likely experienced a few ups and downs along the journey. Soon you'll be planning meals on your own, but this week, you've got nothing to worry about at all. Just enjoy the ride, carefree, and breezy!

If you have some spare time this week, do a quick online search for vegan-friendly restaurants in your area and browse their menu to find dishes you may want to try. As mentioned before, vegan restaurant directories such as *HappyCow* and *VegGuide* are great resources for finding vegan-friendly restaurants. Keep an eye out for Japanese, Thai, Chinese, Mediterranean, and Indian restaurants, which are usually vegan-friendly. Make a list of vegan options for when you're ready to start eating out!

BREAKFAST	LUNCH	SNACK	DINNER
2 **Morning Cereal Bars**, 1 c. orange juice	Sandwich with 1 oz. **Sun-Dried Tomato Pesto** (see recipe in Week 2, Mon.), 1 oz. avocado, ¼ medium tomato, 4 slices cucumber, and ½ c. sprouts on 2 slices whole grain bread	Mixed vegetables (½ cucumber, 2 oz. baby carrots, ½ c. broccoli) with 2 T. hummus	5 oz. **Asian Sesame Tahini Noodles** (see recipe in Week 1, Sat.)

MORNING CEREAL BARS

Yields 14 bars

Store-bought breakfast bars are often loaded with artificial sugars, and most homemade recipes require corn syrup. This healthier method makes a sweet and filling snack or breakfast to munch on the run. Swap in other dried fruits for the raisins if you prefer.

3 c. crispy rice cereal	½ t. vanilla
1 c. peanut butter	2 c. muesli
⅓ c. tahini	½ c. flax meal
1 c. maple syrup	½ c. raisins

1. Lightly grease a baking pan or two casserole pans.
2. Place cereal in a sealable bag and crush partially with a rolling pin. If you're using a smaller cereal, you can skip this step. Set aside.
3. Combine peanut butter, tahini, and maple syrup in a large saucepan over low heat, stirring well to combine.
4. Remove from heat and stir in vanilla, and then cereal, muesli, flax meal, and raisins.
5. Press firmly into greased baking pan and chill until firm, about 45 minutes, then slice into bars.

PER SERVING (1 BAR) Calories **305** Fat **15G** Protein **8G** Sodium **69MG** Fiber **4G** Carbohydrates **40G** Sugar **23G** Zinc **2MG** Calcium **57MG** Iron **4MG** Vit. D **1MCG** Vit. B$_{12}$ **2MCG**

DON'T GET BORED OF BREAD!

Exploring a few quality gourmet ingredients can really perk up your vegan diet if you're in a rut. Use an artisan bread to make sandwiches more satisfying, and leave the regular stuff for morning toast. Try ciabatta rolls, focaccia, or visit your local bakery to try something new.

What I Ate

DATE [   ] | [   ] | [   ]

TIME	FOOD ITEM	AMOUNT	CALORIES	FAT	CARBS	FIBER	PROTEIN
	TOTAL						

Today's Vegan Plate

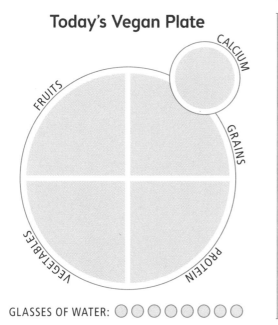

CALCIUM

FRUITS

GRAINS

VEGETABLES

PROTEIN

GLASSES OF WATER: ○○○○○○○○

Thoughts about Today

MENU

BREAKFAST	LUNCH	SNACK	DINNER
1 c. instant grits with 1 (1-oz.) slice vegan cheese, 1 c. unsweetened applesauce	1 baked potato with ½ c. black beans, ⅓ c. salsa, and 1 oz. vegan cheese; side green salad with 2 c. romaine lettuce, 1 tomato, and 1 diced cucumber, and 2 T. Goddess Dressing (see recipe in Week 1, Mon.)	Mixed fruit salad with ½ apple, ½ banana, ½ c. strawberries, and ½ c. pineapple	4 oz. Lazy and Hungry Garlic Pasta with 1 diced tomato and 1 slice of garlic bread

LAZY AND HUNGRY GARLIC PASTA

Serves 6

Simple to make and mouthwatering to eat—this recipe is a double threat! Serve with garlic bread, if desired.

2 cloves garlic, minced	½ t. dried parsley
2 T. olive oil	⅛ t. red pepper flakes
3 c. pasta, cooked	1 t. salt
2 T. nutritional yeast	1 t. black pepper

1. Heat garlic in olive oil for just 1–2 minutes until almost browned.
2. Toss garlic and olive oil with remaining ingredients.

PER SERVING Calories **166** Fat **5G** Protein **5G** Sodium **489MG** Fiber **2G** Carbohydrates **24G** Sugar **0G** Zinc **1MG** Calcium **10MG** Iron **1MG** Vit. D **0MCG** Vit. B_{12} **1MCG**

THE PERFECT VEGAN FLAVOR MIX?

Garlic powder, nutritional yeast, and salt is a delicious seasoning combination, and will give you a bit of B_{11} perk-up. Perfect for vegans. Use it over toast, vegetables, popcorn, bagels, baked potatoes, and of course, cooked pasta, if you're feeling, well, lazy and hungry!

What I Ate

DATE [   ] | [   ] | [   ]

TIME	FOOD ITEM	AMOUNT	CALORIES	FAT	CARBS	FIBER	PROTEIN
		TOTAL					

Today's Vegan Plate

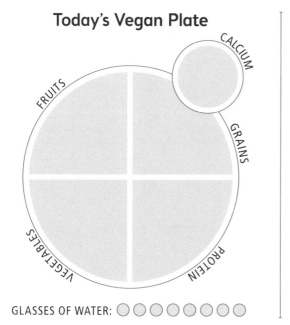

GLASSES OF WATER: ○○○○○○○○

Thoughts about Today

MENU

BREAKFAST	LUNCH	SNACK	DINNER
1 c. whole grain cereal with ½ c. oat milk	1 vegan grilled cheese sandwich with 2 (1-oz.) slices vegan cheese on 2 slices whole grain bread, 1 c. tomato soup, 1 apple	2 rice cakes with 1 T. almond butter	5 oz. **Basic Baked Tempeh Patties**, 1 c. steamed cauliflower or broccoli, 1 medium baked sweet potato

BASIC BAKED TEMPEH PATTIES

Serves 2

Baked tempeh is a simple entrée, or you can use it as a patty to make veggie burgers or sandwiches. Slice your tempeh into cubes to add to fried rice, noodles, or stir-fries. Tofurky makes a premarinated sliced tempeh, perfect for when you're in a pinch.

1 (8-oz.) package tempeh
1 c. plus 2 T. water, divided
3 T. soy sauce
2 T. apple cider vinegar
3 cloves garlic, minced
2 t. sesame oil

1. If your tempeh is thicker than ¾", slice in half through the center to make 2 thinner pieces, then cut into desired shapes.
2. Simmer tempeh in 1 cup water for 10 minutes; drain well.
3. Whisk together remaining ingredients, including 2 tablespoons water, and marinate tempeh for at least 1 hour or overnight.
4. Preheat oven to 375°F and transfer tempeh to a lightly greased baking sheet.
5. Bake for 10–12 minutes on each side.

PER SERVING Calories 498 Fat 29G Protein 48G Sodium 1,340MG Fiber 0G Carbohydrates 20G Sugar 0G Zinc 3MG Calcium 269MG Iron 7MG Vit. D 0MCG Vit. B$_{12}$ 0MCG

USING "PLANNED-OVERS"

Cooked whole grains can stretch out just about any meal to add some healthy fiber and a touch of homemade goodness to canned chili and soup, baked beans, and even green salads or bean salads. Whenever you cook grains, cook a cup or so extra and store them in the refrigerator. When stored properly in a tightly sealed container, grains can keep for 3–4 days in the fridge. Your future self will thank you!

What I Ate

DATE _____ | _____ | _____

TIME	FOOD ITEM	AMOUNT	CALORIES	FAT	CARBS	FIBER	PROTEIN
TOTAL							

Today's Vegan Plate

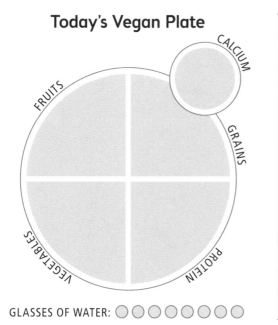

CALCIUM

FRUITS

GRAINS

VEGETABLES

PROTEIN

GLASSES OF WATER: ○○○○○○○○

Thoughts about Today

MENU

BREAKFAST	LUNCH	SNACK	DINNER
1 bagel with 2 T. hummus or vegan cream cheese, 1 c. oat milk	Eggless Egg Salad (see recipe in Week 4, Mon.) sandwich with ¼ tomato (sliced) and ¼ c. kale on 2 slices whole grain bread	Mixed fruit salad with ½ apple, ½ banana, ½ c. strawberries, and ½ c. pineapple; 1 oz. raisins	9¼ oz. Eggplant Baba Ganoush; 1 pita; and Greek spinach salad with 2 c. fresh spinach, ½ red bell pepper, 2 T. black olives, ¼ c. chopped artichoke hearts, and 2 T. Goddess Dressing (see recipe in Week 1, Mon.)

EGGPLANT BABA GANOUSH

Serves 4

If you've never had baba ganoush before, get ready to be blown away by this tasty Middle Eastern classic.

2 medium eggplants	½ t. cumin
3 T. olive oil, divided	½ t. chili powder
2 T. lemon juice	¼ t. salt
¼ c. tahini	1 T. chopped fresh parsley
3 cloves garlic, minced	

1. Preheat oven to 400°F. Slice eggplants in half and prick several times with a fork.
2. Place on a baking sheet and drizzle with 1 tablespoon olive oil. Bake for 30 minutes, turning once halfway through. Allow to cool slightly.
3. Remove inner flesh and place in a bowl.
4. Using a large fork or potato masher, mash eggplant together with remaining ingredients until almost smooth.

PER SERVING Calories 254 Fat 19G Protein 6G Sodium 167MG Fiber 8G Carbohydrates 21G Sugar 9G Zinc 1MG Calcium 55MG Iron 2MG Vit. D 0MCG Vit. B$_{12}$ 0MCG

HALFWAY HOMEMADE VEGAN MEALS

Shop the ethnic food aisle or bulk section for mixes that can be prepared at home in an instant. Tabouli, hummus, and falafel mixes and even veggie burger mixes are a great thing to keep on hand. Just add water or olive oil, and they're ready to go. To freshen them up a bit, mix a few fresh tomatoes into a tabouli mix, or add in some sliced olives or cumin to a hummus mix.

What I Ate

DATE [   ] | [   ] | [   ]

TIME	FOOD ITEM	AMOUNT	CALORIES	FAT	CARBS	FIBER	PROTEIN
	TOTAL						

Today's Vegan Plate

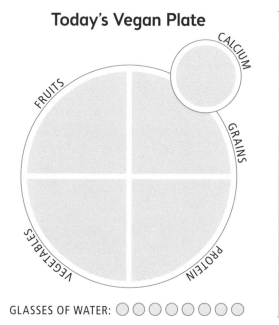

GLASSES OF WATER: ○○○○○○○○

Thoughts about Today

MENU

BREAKFAST	LUNCH	SNACK	DINNER
1 c. baked beans, 2 slices whole grain toast, 1 banana, 1 c. chocolate soy milk	9¼ oz. leftover **Eggplant Baba Ganoush** (see recipe in Week 9, Thurs.); 1 pita; side green salad with 2 c. romaine lettuce, 1 tomato, and 1 diced cucumber, and 2 T. **Goddess Dressing** (see recipe in Week 1, Mon.); 1 c. tomato juice (no salt added)	1 apple, 1 T. peanut butter, 1 oz. raisins	Vegan chicken burger with 1 vegan chicken patty, ¼ tomato (sliced), ¼ c. of romaine lettuce, 1 T. vegan mayonnaise, and 12.5 oz. **Sesame and Soy Cole Slaw Salad**

SESAME AND SOY COLE SLAW SALAD

Serves 2

This colorful twist on traditional slaw is perfect for a get-together or potluck.

1 medium head Napa cabbage, shredded	2 T. olive oil
1 medium carrot, grated	2 T. apple cider vinegar
2 scallions, chopped	2 t. soy sauce
1 medium red bell pepper, sliced thin	½ t. sesame oil
	2 T. maple syrup
	2 T. sesame seeds

1. Toss together cabbage, carrot, scallions, and bell pepper in a large bowl.
2. In a separate small bowl, whisk together olive oil, vinegar, soy sauce, sesame oil, and maple syrup until well combined.
3. Drizzle dressing over cabbage and vegetables, add sesame seeds, and toss well to combine.

PER SERVING Calories **343** Fat **20G** Protein **9G** Sodium **394MG** Fiber **7G** Carbohydrates **38G** Sugar **23G** Zinc **2MG** Calcium **342MG** Iron **4MG** Vit. D **0MCG** Vit. B$_{12}$ **0MCG**

MIDEAST TREATS

Middle Eastern restaurants are always a safe bet for vegans eating out. You're almost always guaranteed to find vegan falafel, hummus, baba ganoush, fattoush, and those absolutely divine stuffed grape leaves. The best part? They're all vegan already! No need to ask a server to hold the cheese.

What I Ate

DATE [   ] | [   ] | [   ]

TIME	FOOD ITEM	AMOUNT	CALORIES	FAT	CARBS	FIBER	PROTEIN
		TOTAL					

Today's Vegan Plate

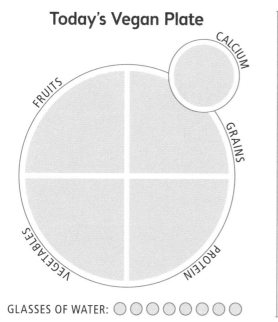

CALCIUM
FRUITS
GRAINS
VEGETABLES
PROTEIN

Thoughts about Today

GLASSES OF WATER: ○○○○○○○○

MENU

BREAKFAST	LUNCH	SNACK	DINNER
3 slices **Easy Vegan French Toast** (see recipe in Week 1, Sun.), 1 c. fresh strawberries, 1 c. orange juice	3 oz. **Lemon Quinoa Veggie Salad**	1 c. edamame	12 oz. **Polenta and Chili Casserole**, 1 c. steamed spinach with 16g nutritional yeast

LEMON QUINOA VEGGIE SALAD

Serves 6

Adding vegetables to protein-packed quinoa makes this dish a nutritional home run.

1½ c. quinoa	¼ c. olive oil
4 c. vegetable broth	1 t. garlic powder
1 c. frozen mixed vegetables, thawed	½ t. sea salt
	¼ t. black pepper
¼ c. lemon juice	2 T. chopped fresh parsley

1. In a large pot, simmer quinoa in vegetable broth for 15–20 minutes, stirring occasionally until liquid is absorbed and quinoa is cooked. Add mixed vegetables and stir to combine.
2. Remove from heat and combine with remaining ingredients. Serve hot or cold.

PER SERVING Calories **264** Fat **12G** Protein **7G** Sodium **715MG** Fiber **4G** Carbohydrates **33G** Sugar **3G** Zinc **2MG** Calcium **35MG** Iron **2MG** Vit. D **0MCG** Vit. B$_{12}$ **0MG**

POLENTA AND CHILI CASSEROLE

Serves 6

Using canned chili and thawed frozen vegetables, you can get this quick one-pot casserole meal in the oven in just about 10 minutes.

3 (14.7-oz.) cans vegan chili (or about 6 c. homemade)	1 c. cornmeal
	2½ c. water
	2 T. vegan margarine
2 c. diced frozen mixed vegetables, thawed and drained	1 T. chili powder

1. Combine vegan chili and vegetables, and spread in the bottom of a lightly greased casserole dish.
2. Preheat oven to 375°F.
3. Over low heat, combine cornmeal and water. Simmer, stirring frequently, for 10 minutes. Stir in vegan margarine.
4. Spread cornmeal mixture over chili and sprinkle the top with chili powder.
5. Bake uncovered for 20–25 minutes.

PER SERVING Calories **356** Fat **7G** Protein **18G** Sodium **927MG** Fiber **12G** Carbohydrates **57G** Sugar **2G** Zinc **1MG** Calcium **141MG** Iron **7MG** Vit. D **0MCG** Vit. B$_{12}$ **0MCG**

What I Ate

DATE | |

TIME	FOOD ITEM	AMOUNT	CALORIES	FAT	CARBS	FIBER	PROTEIN
	TOTAL						

Today's Vegan Plate

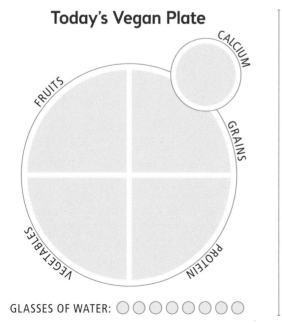

GLASSES OF WATER: ○ ○ ○ ○ ○ ○ ○ ○

Thoughts about Today

MENU

BREAKFAST	LUNCH	SNACK	DINNER
1 c. **Pumpkin Protein Smoothie** (see recipe in Week 3, Thurs.), 1 banana, 1 oz. cashews	Bean burrito with ½ c. beef substitute, 1 large flour tortilla, ½ tomato (sliced), ½ chopped onion, and ½ c. iceberg lettuce	1 **Peanut Butter Rice Crispies**	¼ block **Easy Barbecue Baked Tofu** (see recipe in Week 2, Wed.), 1 c. **Caramelized Baby Carrots** (see recipe in Week 1, Tues.), 1 ear corn on the cob

PEANUT BUTTER RICE CRISPIES

Serves 9

These sticky treats will be a hit at the school bake sale or a special dinner.

¾ c. sugar
¾ c. golden syrup
¾ c. peanut butter

4½ c. crispy rice cereal
⅔ c. chocolate chips

1. Lightly grease a 9" × 9" baking dish.
2. Heat sugar and golden syrup on the stove top just until simmering. Remove from heat and stir in peanut butter until well combined, then gently stir in cereal and chocolate chips.
3. Spread mixture evenly into baking pan, using a large spoon or spatula to flatten. Chill in the refrigerator until firm, then slice into squares.

PER SERVING Calories **360** Fat **15G** Protein **7G** Sodium **129MG** Fiber **3G** Carbohydrates **56G** Sugar **42G** Zinc **1MG** Calcium **18MG** Iron **5MG** Vit. D **1MCG** Vit. B$_{12}$ **1MCG**

HONEY: TO BEE OR NOT TO BEE?

Many vegans assume honey is cruelty-free and gently collected from bees that are producing it naturally, but like all animals, bees want to live their lives free from harm. The honeybee population is declining at alarming rates due to disease, pesticides, and climate change. Though the subject is often debated among vegans, according to the manifesto set forth by the British Vegan Society in 1944, honey is an animal by-product and therefore not vegan. Agave nectar, maple syrup, organic cane sugar, molasses, sorghum, just to name a few, can easily replace honey in recipes. Vegan lip balms and bee wax–free candles can be found at your local health food store.

What I Ate

DATE [ ] | [ ] | [ ]

TIME	FOOD ITEM	AMOUNT	CALORIES	FAT	CARBS	FIBER	PROTEIN
TOTAL							

Today's Vegan Plate

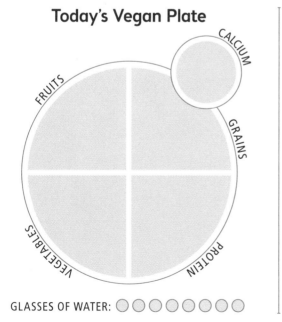

CALCIUM

FRUITS

GRAINS

VEGETABLES

PROTEIN

GLASSES OF WATER: ○○○○○○○○○

Thoughts about Today

REVIEW

I FEEL:

_____
_____
_____
_____

MY GREATEST FOOD DISCOVERY THIS WEEK WAS:

_____
_____
_____
_____

THIS WEEK'S BIGGEST VEGAN CHALLENGE WAS:

_____
_____
_____
_____

NEW FOOD I'D LIKE TO TRY:

_____
_____
_____
_____

WHEN I LOOK BACK AT THIS WEEK, I MOST WANT TO REMEMBER:

_____
_____
_____

HOW ARE YOU PROGRESSING TOWARD YOUR GOALS?

_____
_____
_____
_____

WEEK 10

You're already at Week 10! Now is a great time to start planning how you'll be eating after these twelve weeks are up. Are there some meals that you loved and will continue eating every week? Or perhaps you never want to touch tempeh ever again? Identify a few convenience foods that will keep you well stocked and well fed under any circumstances. Start collecting a few recipes that you'd like to try once you're on your own, and maybe even plan a few complete meals to have on deck ready to go for Week 13. Meals don't have to be complex to be nutritious. Think of a few things you can make easily, without a recipe. Chickpeas with a few tomatoes and Indian spices paired with quinoa can be on your plate in minutes. Beans can be simmered with chili powder and paired with rice and vegetables. A huge vegetable salad is always delicious and easy to make. Think you can whip up some vegan burritos, tacos, soups, and tofu dishes without a recipe? You can do this!

Review your notes from the past weeks, and think about some of the meals that you enjoyed and were easy enough to prepare on busy weeknights.

MENU

BREAKFAST	LUNCH	SNACK	DINNER
12 oz. **Chocolate Peanut Butter Banana Smoothie** (see recipe in Week 1, Thurs.)	Barbecue tofu sandwiches with ¼ block leftover **Easy Barbecue Baked Tofu** (see recipe in Week 2, Wed.), ¼ tomato, ¼ c. iceberg lettuce, and 1 T. vegan mayonnaise on 2 slices whole wheat bread; 1 apple or 1 c. grapes	1 **Peanut Butter Rice Crispies** (see recipe in Week 9, Sun.)	10½ oz. **Winter Seitan Stew**; 1 c. steamed cauliflower with 16g nutritional yeast; side green salad with 2 c. romaine lettuce, 1 tomato, 1 diced cucumber, and 2 T. **Goddess Dressing** (see recipe in Week 1, Mon.)

WINTER SEITAN STEW

Serves 6

If you're used to a "meat and potatoes" kind of diet, this hearty seitan and potato stew ought to become a favorite.

2 c. chopped seitan
1 medium onion, chopped
2 medium carrots, chopped
2 stalks celery, chopped
2 T. olive oil
4 c. vegetable broth

2 medium russet potatoes, chopped
½ t. dried sage
½ t. dried rosemary
½ t. dried thyme
2 T. cornstarch
⅓ c. water
1 t. salt
1 t. black pepper

1. In a large soup pot, heat seitan, onion, carrots, and celery in olive oil, for 4–5 minutes, stirring frequently until seitan is lightly browned.
2. Add vegetable broth and potatoes and bring to a boil. Reduce to a simmer, add spices and cover. Allow to cook for 25–30 minutes until potatoes are soft.
3. In a small bowl, whisk together cornstarch and water. Add to soup, stirring to combine.
4. Cook, uncovered, for another 5–7 minutes until stew has thickened.
5. Season with salt and pepper.

PER SERVING Calories **221** Fat **5G** Protein **17G** Sodium **1,101MG** Fiber **3G** Carbohydrates **29G** Sugar **4G** Zinc **0MG** Calcium **75MG** Iron **3MG** Vit. D **0MCG** Vit. B$_{12}$ **0MCG**

WHAT ARE ANIMAL RIGHTS?

Philosophers Jeremy Bentham and Peter Singer have both written about dominance, use, and exploitation of one being (animals) by another (humans) as a reason to reject animal foods, a concept known as *speciesism*. The words of novelist, feminist, and vegan Alice Walker summarize this sentiment: "The animals of the world exist for their own reasons. They were not made for humans any more than black people were made for white, or women created for men." This is the idea of animal rights, that animals may lead their own lives, completely unencumbered by humans.

What I Ate

DATE ▢ | ▢ | ▢

TIME	FOOD ITEM	AMOUNT	CALORIES	FAT	CARBS	FIBER	PROTEIN
TOTAL							

Today's Vegan Plate

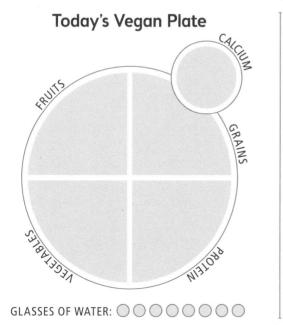

FRUITS

CALCIUM

GRAINS

VEGETABLES

PROTEIN

GLASSES OF WATER: ◯◯◯◯◯◯◯◯

Thoughts about Today

MENU

BREAKFAST	LUNCH	SNACK	DINNER
1 c. oatmeal with 2 t. maple syrup, 1 oz. pecans, 1 c. blueberries	7 oz. leftover Winter Seitan Stew (see recipe in Week 10, Mon.), 1 slice whole grain toast, 1 c. orange juice	Mixed vegetables (½ cucumber, 2 oz. baby carrots, ½ c. broccoli) in 2 T. hummus	5 oz. Sloppy "Jolindas" with TVP, baked sweet potato, and 16g nutritional yeast; side green salad with 2 c. romaine lettuce, 1 tomato, 1 diced cucumber, and 2 T. Goddess Dressing (see recipe in Week 1, Mon.)

SLOPPY "JOLINDAS" WITH TVP

Serves 8

TVP "Sloppy Jolindas" are reminiscent of those goopy sloppy joes served up in primary school cafeterias, with all of the nostalgic comfort and none of the gristle or mystery meat. The TVP is only partially rehydrated, the better to absorb all the flavors.

1¾ c. TVP
1 c. hot water
1 medium onion, chopped
1 medium green bell pepper, chopped small
2 T. vegetable oil
1 (16-oz.) can tomato sauce
¼ c. barbecue sauce
2 T. chili powder
1 T. mustard powder
1 T. soy sauce
2 T. molasses
2 T. apple cider vinegar
1 t. hot sauce
1 t. garlic powder
½ t. salt

1. Combine TVP and water and allow to sit at least 5 minutes.
2. In a large soup or stockpot, sauté onion and bell pepper in oil until soft.
3. Reduce heat to medium low and add TVP and remaining ingredients. Simmer, covered, for at least 15 minutes, stirring occasionally.
4. For thicker and less sloppy "Sloppy Jolindas," simmer a bit longer, uncovered, to reduce the liquid.

PER SERVING Calories 164 Fat 4G Protein 12G Sodium 678MG Fiber 6G Carbohydrates 20G Sugar 13G Zinc 0MG Calcium 105MG Iron 4MG Vit. D 0MCG Vit. B$_{12}$ 0MCG

YEAST EXTRACTS

Yeast extracts such as Marmite and Vegemite are more popular abroad than in the United States, and most people tend to either love them or hate them. If you've never tried them, there's only one way to find out how you feel! Both are a great source of B vitamins for vegans. Try spreading a bit of yeast extract on your toast, or have a peanut butter and Marmite sandwich! Most people are pretty loyal to one brand or the other, so try them both.

What I Ate

DATE [ ] | [ ] | [ ]

TIME	FOOD ITEM	AMOUNT	CALORIES	FAT	CARBS	FIBER	PROTEIN
TOTAL							

Today's Vegan Plate

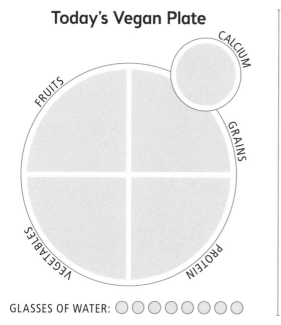

GLASSES OF WATER: ○○○○○○○○○

Thoughts about Today

MENU

BREAKFAST	LUNCH	SNACK	DINNER
1 slice of panfried polenta with ½ c. black beans and 1 (1-oz.) slice vegan cheese, 1 c. almond milk	Leftover Sloppy "Jolindas" with TVP (see recipe in Week 10, Tues.); side green salad with 2 c. romaine lettuce, 1 tomato, 1 diced cucumber, and 2 T. Goddess Dressing (see recipe in Week 1, Mon.)	1 c. edamame, 1 c. strawberries	6 oz. Spicy Southern Jambalaya, 1 vegan sausage patty, 1 c. steamed spinach

SPICY SOUTHERN JAMBALAYA

Serves 6

Make this spicy and smoky Southern rice dish a main meal by adding in some browned mock sausage or sautéed tofu.

1 medium onion, chopped	3 c. water
1 medium bell pepper, any color, chopped	2 c. long grain white rice
	1 bay leaf
1 stalk celery, diced	1 t. paprika
2 T. olive oil	½ t. dried thyme
1 (14-oz.) can diced tomatoes (do not drain)	½ t. dried oregano
	½ t. garlic powder
	1 c. corn
	½ t. hot Tabasco sauce

1. In a large skillet or stockpot, heat onion, bell pepper, and celery in olive oil until almost soft, about 3 minutes.
2. Reduce heat and add remaining ingredients, except corn and hot sauce. Cover, bring to a low simmer, and cook for 20 minutes until rice is done, stirring occasionally.
3. Add corn and hot sauce, and cook just until heated through, about 3 minutes.

PER SERVING Calories 356 Fat 5G Protein 7G Sodium 131MG Fiber 3G Carbohydrates 70G Sugar 6G Zinc 1MG Calcium 41MG Iron 4MG Vit. D 0MCG Vit. B$_{12}$ 0MCG

LEFTOVER RICE

Don't let it go to waste! Use leftover rice to make rice and bean burritos, rice salads, or Asian-style fried rice. Add it to soups or pair it with a stir-fry. Also, leftover plain white rice makes for an excellent rice pudding.

What I Ate

DATE [   ] | [   ] | [   ]

TIME	FOOD ITEM	AMOUNT	CALORIES	FAT	CARBS	FIBER	PROTEIN
		TOTAL					

Today's Vegan Plate

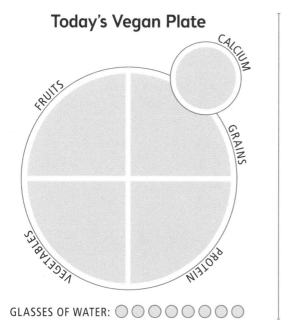

GLASSES OF WATER: ○○○○○○○○

Thoughts about Today

BREAKFAST	LUNCH	SNACK	DINNER
1 c. whole grain cereal with ½ c. soy milk, 1 banana or 1 c. strawberries	6 oz. leftover Spicy Southern Jambalaya (see recipe in Week 10, Wed.) with 1 vegan sausage patty	200 calories of whole grain crackers with 3 T. olive tapenade	6 oz. Tofu BBQ Sauce "Steaks," 4 oz. Baked Sweet Potato Fries (see recipe in Week 4, Thurs.), 1 c. oven-roasted butternut squash

TOFU BBQ SAUCE "STEAKS"

Serves 5

These chewy tofu "steaks" have a hearty texture and a meaty flavor. Delicious as is, or add it to a sandwich.

⅓ c. barbecue sauce	2 (14-oz.) blocks firm or extra-firm tofu, well pressed
¼ c. water	
2 t. balsamic vinegar	½ medium onion, chopped
2 T. soy sauce	2 T. olive oil
1 T. hot sauce (or to taste)	

1. In a small bowl, whisk together barbecue sauce, water, vinegar, soy sauce, and hot sauce until well combined. Set aside.
2. Slice pressed tofu into ¼"-thick strips.
3. Sauté onions in oil, and carefully add tofu. Fry tofu on both sides until lightly golden brown, about 2 minutes on each side.
4. Reduce heat and add barbecue sauce mixture, stirring to coat tofu well. Cook over medium-low heat until sauce absorbs and thickens, about 5–6 minutes.

PER SERVING Calories **222** Fat **13G** Protein **15G** Sodium **545MG** Fiber **2G** Carbohydrates **13G** Sugar **7G** Zinc **0MG** Calcium **210MG** Iron **2MG** Vit. D **0MCG** Vit. B$_{12}$ **0MCG**

TOFU, TEMPEH, AND SEITAN

This recipe, like many panfried tofu recipes, will also work well with seitan or tempeh, though seitan needs a bit longer to cook all the way through; otherwise it ends up tough and chewy.

What I Ate

DATE ___ | ___ | ___

TIME	FOOD ITEM	AMOUNT	CALORIES	FAT	CARBS	FIBER	PROTEIN
TOTAL							

Today's Vegan Plate

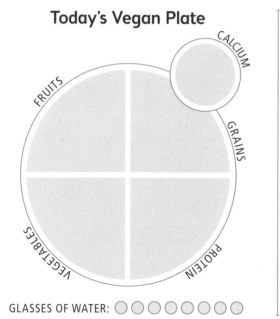

GLASSES OF WATER: ○○○○○○○○

Thoughts about Today

MENU

BREAKFAST	LUNCH	SNACK	DINNER
¾ c. Maple Cinnamon Breakfast Quinoa Bowl (see recipe in Week 4, Fri.)	275 calories store-bought vegan chili; mixed fruit salad with ½ apple, ½ banana, ½ c. strawberries, and ½ c. pineapple; 1 c. orange juice	4 oz. leftover Baked Sweet Potato Fries (see recipe in Week 4, Thurs.), 1 oz. peanuts	8 oz. Italian Veggie and Pasta Casserole, 1 c. steamed broccoli with 16g nutritional yeast

ITALIAN VEGGIE AND PASTA CASSEROLE

Serves 8

Vegetables and pasta are baked into an Italian-spiced casserole with a crumbly topping. Add in a handful of TVP crumbles or some kidney beans if you want a protein boost.

1 (16-oz.) package pasta (use a medium pasta like bow ties, cork-screws, or small shells)

1 medium onion, chopped

3 medium zucchinis, sliced

1 medium red bell pepper, chopped

4 cloves garlic, minced

2 T. olive oil

1 (28-oz.) can diced tomatoes

¾ c. corn kernels

1 t. dried parsley

1 t. dried basil

½ t. dried oregano

½ t. crushed red pepper flakes

¼ t. black pepper

1 c. bread crumbs

½ c. grated vegan cheese

1. Cook pasta according to package instructions, drain well, and layer in a baking dish.
2. Preheat oven to 425°F.
3. Sauté onion, zucchini, bell pepper, and garlic in olive oil just until soft, about 3–4 minutes. Add tomatoes, corn, parsley, basil, oregano, and crushed red pepper. Simmer for 8–10 minutes and season with black pepper.
4. Cover pasta with zucchini and tomato mixture. Sprinkle with bread crumbs and vegan cheese.
5. Bake for 10–12 minutes.

PER SERVING Calories 409 Fat 9G Protein 13G Sodium 608MG Fiber 7G Carbohydrates 70G Sugar 9G Zinc 2MG Calcium 99MG Iron 4MG Vit. D 0MCG Vit. B$_{12}$ 0MCG

What I Ate

DATE [ ] | [ ] | [ ]

TIME	FOOD ITEM	AMOUNT	CALORIES	FAT	CARBS	FIBER	PROTEIN
TOTAL							

Today's Vegan Plate

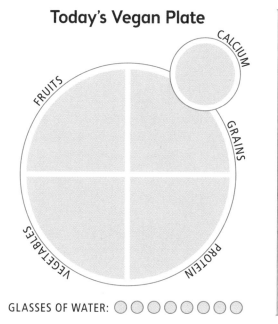

FRUITS

CALCIUM

GRAINS

VEGETABLES

PROTEIN

GLASSES OF WATER: ○ ○ ○ ○ ○ ○ ○ ○

Thoughts about Today

BREAKFAST	LUNCH	SNACK	DINNER
3 Vegan Pancakes (see recipe in Week 3, Sun.), 1 c. fresh strawberries, 1 c. orange juice	6 oz. Mexico City Protein Bowl	1 c. plant-based yogurt with ⅓ c. granola	1½ c. Barley Vegetable Soup; side green salad with 2 c. romaine lettuce, 1 tomato, 1 diced cucumber, and 2 T. Goddess Dressing (see recipe in Week 1, Mon.)

MEXICO CITY PROTEIN BOWL

Serves 4

This flavor-packed bowl will have you looking for flights to Mexico! Top with vegan sour cream, if desired (try Tofutti's Sour Cream or Vegan Gourmet's Sour Cream).

½ (14-oz.) block firm tofu, diced small
1 scallion, chopped
1 T. olive oil
½ c. peas
½ c. corn kernels
½ t. chili powder
1 (15-oz.) can black beans, drained
2 large corn tortillas
1 medium avocado, sliced
1 medium tomato, diced
1 t. hot sauce

1. Heat tofu and scallion in olive oil for 2–3 minutes, then add peas, corn, and chili powder. Cook another 1–2 minutes, stirring frequently.
2. Reduce heat to medium low, and add black beans. Heat for 4–5 minutes until well combined and heated through.
3. Place 2 corn tortillas in the bottom of a bowl, and spoon beans, avocado, diced tomato, and tofu over the top. Season with hot sauce.

PER SERVING Calories 289 Fat 14G Protein 13G Sodium 206MG Fiber 10G Carbohydrates 31G Sugar 3G Zinc 1MG Calcium 141MG Iron 3MG Vit. D 0MCG Vit. B₁₂ 0MCG

BARLEY VEGETABLE SOUP

Serves 6

Barley and vegetable soup is an excellent "kitchen sink" recipe, meaning that you can toss in just about any fresh or frozen vegetables or spices you happen to have on hand.

1 medium onion, chopped
2 medium carrots, sliced
2 stalks celery, chopped
2 T. olive oil
8 c. vegetable broth
1 c. barley
1½ c. frozen mixed vegetables
1 (14-oz.) can crushed or diced tomatoes
½ t. dried parsley
½ t. dried thyme
2 bay leaves
1 t. salt
1 t. black pepper

1. In a large soup or stockpot, sauté onion, carrots, and celery in olive oil for 3–5 minutes, just until onion is almost soft.
2. Reduce heat to medium low, and add remaining ingredients, except salt and pepper.
3. Bring to a simmer, cover, and allow to cook for at least 45 minutes, stirring occasionally.
4. Remove cover and allow to cook for 10 more minutes.
5. Remove bay leaves, season with salt and pepper.

PER SERVING Calories 239 Fat 5G Protein 7G Sodium 1,535MG Fiber 10G Carbohydrates 44G Sugar 8G Zinc 1MG Calcium 72MG Iron 2MG Vit. D 0MCG Vit. B₁₂ 0MCG

What I Ate

DATE [   ] | [   ] | [   ]

TIME	FOOD ITEM	AMOUNT	CALORIES	FAT	CARBS	FIBER	PROTEIN
TOTAL							

Today's Vegan Plate

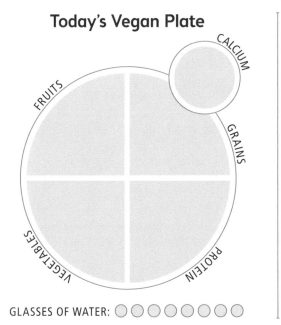

CALCIUM

FRUITS

GRAINS

VEGETABLES

PROTEIN

GLASSES OF WATER: ○○○○○○○○○

Thoughts about Today

MENU

BREAKFAST	LUNCH	SNACK	DINNER
¾ c. frozen hash browns (about 250 calories) with ½ c. black beans, 1 oz. vegan cheese, 1 c. orange juice	1½ c. leftover **Barley Vegetable Soup** (see recipe in Week 10, Sat.), 1 slice whole grain toast, 1 banana	2 **Easy Banana Date Cookies**, 1 apple or 1 pear	**Saucy Kung Pao Tofu** with ½ c. brown rice

EASY BANANA DATE COOKIES

Yields 1 dozen

Even store-bought vegan cookies can lack in nutrition. Try these instead—the dates and banana make them healthy as well as delicious.

1 c. chopped, pitted dates   ¼ t. vanilla
Water for soaking   1¾ c. coconut flakes
1 medium banana, ripe

1. Preheat oven to 375°F.
2. Cover dates in water, and soak for about 10 minutes until softened. Drain.
3. Process together dates, banana, and vanilla until almost smooth.
4. Stir in coconut flakes by hand until thick. You may need a little more or less than 1¾ cups.
5. Drop by large tablespoonfuls onto ungreased baking sheet, and bake 10–12 minutes or until done. Cookies will be soft and chewy.

PER SERVING (1 COOKIE) Calories **85** Fat **4G** Protein **1G** Sodium **3MG** Fiber **2G** Carbohydrates **13G** Sugar **10G** Zinc **0MG** Calcium **7MG** Iron **0MG** Vit. D **0MCG** Vit. B$_{12}$ **0MCG**

SAUCY KUNG PAO TOFU

Serves 6

Skip the takeout and make your own version of this dish. Serve over cooked white rice.

3 T. soy sauce
2 T. rice vinegar
1 T. sesame oil
2 (14-oz.) blocks extra-firm tofu
1 medium red bell pepper, chopped
1 medium green bell pepper, chopped
1 c. fresh baby corn
⅔ c. sliced button mushrooms
3 cloves garlic, minced
3 small chili peppers, diced
1 t. red pepper flakes
2 T. olive oil
1 t. ginger powder
½ c. water
½ t. sugar
1½ t. cornstarch
2 scallions, chopped
½ c. peanuts

1. Whisk together soy sauce, rice vinegar, and sesame oil in a shallow pan or zip-lock bag. Add tofu, and marinate for at least 1 hour; the longer, the better. Drain tofu, reserving marinade.
2. Sauté bell peppers, corn, mushrooms, garlic, chili peppers, and red pepper flakes in olive oil for 2–3 minutes, then add tofu, and heat for another 1–2 minutes until vegetables are almost soft.
3. Reduce heat to medium low, and add marinade, ginger powder, water, sugar, and cornstarch, whisking in the cornstarch to avoid lumps.
4. Heat a few more minutes, stirring constantly until sauce has almost thickened.
5. Add scallions and peanuts, and heat for 1 more minute.

PER SERVING Calories **277** Fat **18G** Protein **17G** Sodium **450MG** Fiber **4G** Carbohydrates **15G** Sugar **4G** Zinc **1MG** Calcium **188MG** Iron **2MG** Vit. D **0MCG** Vit. B$_{12}$ **0MCG**

What I Ate

DATE ⬚ | ⬚ | ⬚

TIME	FOOD ITEM	AMOUNT	CALORIES	FAT	CARBS	FIBER	PROTEIN
		TOTAL					

Today's Vegan Plate

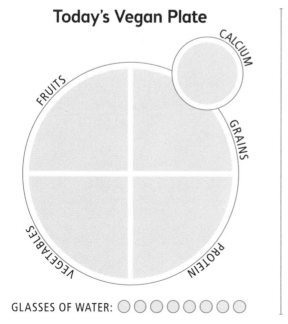

GLASSES OF WATER: ⚪⚪⚪⚪⚪⚪⚪⚪

Thoughts about Today

REVIEW

I FEEL:

MY GREATEST FOOD DISCOVERY THIS WEEK WAS:

THIS WEEK'S BIGGEST VEGAN CHALLENGE WAS:

NEW FOOD I'D LIKE TO TRY:

WHEN I LOOK BACK AT THIS WEEK, I MOST WANT TO REMEMBER:

HOW ARE YOU PROGRESSING TOWARD YOUR GOALS?

WEEK 11

You're comfortable eating vegan, but have you considered veganizing the rest of your life? Start with the kitchen. Open up your cupboards and take a look. What's in your dish soap, laundry detergent, and kitchen cleaners? Are they full of chemicals? Tested on animals? Time to switch to something gentler on you, the animals, and Mother Earth. Make a note to pick up some natural cleaning products next time you make a grocery store run. Next, take a look at the bathroom and the rest of your house. If your shampoos, cosmetics, and personal products are full of harsh chemicals, consider replacing them with organic, cruelty-free brands. Be sure to read the labels on your products. If it doesn't say "Not tested on animals" right there on the label, there's a very good chance it is. What a great excuse for a little retail therapy!

Treat yourself to one or two new animal- and earth-friendly personal products this week (you deserve it, of course!), and browse around for a few brands that you'd like to try in the future. If you're unsure where to start, the Internet is a great source for finding out which companies and brands do and don't test on animals.

BREAKFAST	LUNCH	SNACK	DINNER
1 c. whole grain cereal with ½ c. cashew milk	Veggie burger with ¼ tomato (sliced) and ¼ c. kale; mixed fruit salad with ½ apple, ½ banana, ½ c. strawberries, and ½ c. pineapple	1 **Easy Banana Date Cookies** (see recipe in Week 10, Sun.), 1 oz. almonds	10 oz. **Orange Ginger Mixed Veggie Stir-Fry** with 1 c. rice noodles. 1 c. tomato juice (no salt added)

ORANGE GINGER MIXED VEGGIE STIR-FRY

Serves 4

Rice vinegar can be substituted for the apple cider vinegar, if you prefer. As with most stir-fry recipes, the vegetables are merely a suggestion; use your favorites or whatever looks like it's been sitting too long in your crisper.

3 T. orange juice	2 T. olive oil
1 T. apple cider vinegar	1 bunch broccoli, chopped
2 T. soy sauce	½ c. sliced button mushrooms
2 T. water	½ c. snap peas, chopped
1 T. maple syrup	1 medium carrot, sliced
1 t. powdered ginger	1 c. chopped bok choy
2 cloves garlic, minced	

1. Whisk together orange juice, vinegar, soy sauce, water, maple syrup, and powdered ginger.
2. Heat garlic in olive oil and add vegetables. Allow to cook, stirring frequently, over high heat for 2–3 minutes until just starting to get tender.
3. Add sauce and reduce heat. Simmer, stirring frequently, for another 3–4 minutes, or until vegetables are cooked.

PER SERVING Calories **163** Fat **8G** Protein **7G** Sodium **525MG** Fiber **6G** Carbohydrates **21G** Sugar **9G** Zinc **1MG** Calcium **111MG** Iron **2MG** Vit. D **0MCG** Vit. B$_{12}$ **0MCG**

COOKING WITH RICE NOODLES

When stir-frying a saucy vegetable dish, you can add quick-cooking Asian-style noodles right into the pan. Add some extra sauce ingredients and ¼–½ cup of water. Add the noodles, stir up the sauce, reduce the heat so the vegetables don't scald, and keep covered for just a few minutes.

What I Ate

DATE [ ] | [ ] | [ ]

TIME	FOOD ITEM	AMOUNT	CALORIES	FAT	CARBS	FIBER	PROTEIN
		TOTAL					

Today's Vegan Plate

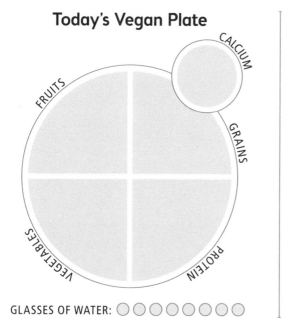

GLASSES OF WATER: ○○○○○○○○

Thoughts about Today

MENU

BREAKFAST	LUNCH	SNACK	DINNER
1 bagel with 2 T. almond butter and 1 sliced banana	10 oz. leftover Orange Ginger Mixed Veggie Stir-Fry (see recipe in Week 11, Mon.) with 1 c. rice noodles, 1 c. orange juice	Mixed vegetables (½ cucumber, 2 oz. baby carrots, ½ c. broccoli) with 2 T. hummus	8 oz. Mexican Rice with Corn and Peppers; ½ c. black beans; side green salad with 2 c. romaine lettuce or a leafy green of your preference, 1 tomato, 1 diced cucumber, and 2 T. Goddess Dressing (see recipe in Week 1, Mon.)

MEXICAN RICE WITH CORN AND PEPPERS

Serves 4

Although Mexican rice is usually served as a side dish, this recipe loads up the vegetables, making it hearty enough for a main dish. Use frozen or canned vegetables if you need to save time.

2 cloves garlic, minced	¼ c. minced Spanish onion
1 c. long-grain white rice	Kernels from 1 ear of corn
2 T. olive oil	1 medium carrot, diced
3 c. vegetable broth	1 t. chili powder
1 c. tomato paste (or 4 large tomatoes, puréed)	½ t. cumin
	¼ t. dried oregano
1 medium green bell pepper, chopped	$\frac{1}{3}$ t. cayenne pepper
	$\frac{1}{3}$ t. salt
1 medium red bell pepper, chopped	1 t. lime juice
	2 t. chopped cilantro

1. Add garlic, rice, and olive oil to a large skillet and heat on medium-high heat, stirring frequently. Toast rice until just golden brown, about 2–3 minutes.
2. Reduce heat and add vegetable broth and remaining ingredients except lemon juice and cilantro.
3. Bring to a simmer, cover, and allow to cook until liquid is absorbed and rice is cooked, about 20–25 minutes, stirring occasionally.
4. Sprinkle rice with lemon juice and garnish with chopped cilantro.

PER SERVING Calories **370** Fat **8G** Protein **9G** Sodium **759MG** Fiber **6G** Carbohydrates **68G** Sugar **14G** Zinc **2MG** Calcium **62MG** Iron **5MG** Vit. D **0MCG** Vit. B$_{12}$ **0MCG**

CONCERNED ABOUT CALCIUM?

Yes, you do need to make sure you get enough calcium as a vegan, but to build strong bones, you need exercise as well as calcium, so vegan or not, diet is only half the question. And as it turns out, we don't need dairy for strong bones. According to NutritionFacts.org, one study involving 100,000 people showed that milk may actually increase bone and hip fracture rates. Reliable vegan sources of calcium include spinach, kale, broccoli, bok choy, soy milk, black-eyed peas, fortified orange juice, tahini, and tofu.

What I Ate

DATE [   ] | [   ] | [   ]

TIME	FOOD ITEM	AMOUNT	CALORIES	FAT	CARBS	FIBER	PROTEIN
	TOTAL						

Today's Vegan Plate

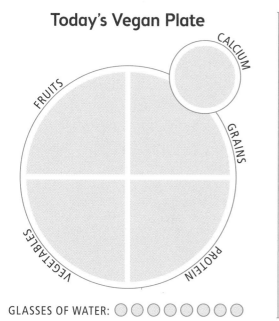

CALCIUM

FRUITS

GRAINS

VEGETABLES

PROTEIN

GLASSES OF WATER: ○ ○ ○ ○ ○ ○ ○ ○

Thoughts about Today

BREAKFAST	LUNCH	SNACK	DINNER
1 vegan sausage patty on an English muffin with 1 (1-oz.) slice vegan cheese, 1 apple	8 oz. leftover Mexican Rice with Corn and Peppers (see recipe in Week 11, Tues.) in a taco shell with 1 oz. vegan cheese, 1 tomato, sliced, ¼ c. iceburg lettuce, 1 c. strawberries	1 oz. almonds with 1 oz. cranberries, 1 pear	Macro-Inspired Veggie Bowl, 1 c. strawberries

MACRO-INSPIRED VEGGIE BOWL

Serves 4

This jam-packed bowl will keep you full for hours! If you don't have Goddess Dressing (see recipe in Week 1, Mon.), serve this with a vegan dressing of your choice.

2 c. cooked brown rice

1 (14-oz.) block baked tofu, chopped into cubes

1 medium head broccoli, chopped and steamed

1 medium red bell pepper, sliced thin

1 (15-oz.) can black beans, drained

1 c. bean sprouts

1 c. Goddess Dressing

½ c. pumpkin seeds

1 medium avocado, sliced

1. Divide brown rice into 4 bowls.
2. Top each bowl with tofu, broccoli, bell pepper, beans, and bean sprouts.
3. Drizzle with dressing, pumpkin seeds, and avocado.

PER SERVING Calories **870** Fat **52G** Protein **41G** Sodium **1,132MG** Fiber **18G** Carbohydrates **69G** Sugar **7G** Zinc **5MG** Calcium **430MG** Iron **9MG** Vit. D **0MCG** Vit. B$_{12}$ **0MCG**

CRAVING HAGGIS?

It's probably not haggis you're going to miss when going vegan, but if it is, there's a vegan substitute! Besides the more common mock chicken and beef products, some of the unbelievable vegan substitutes on the market today include black pudding, vegan caviar, prawns, mutton, and even vegan squid and eel.

What I Ate

DATE | |

TIME	FOOD ITEM	AMOUNT	CALORIES	FAT	CARBS	FIBER	PROTEIN
		TOTAL					

Today's Vegan Plate

CALCIUM

FRUITS

GRAINS

VEGETABLES

PROTEIN

GLASSES OF WATER: ○○○○○○○○

Thoughts about Today

MENU

BREAKFAST	LUNCH	SNACK	DINNER
1 c. Cream of Wheat, 1 banana, 1 c. soy hot chocolate	1½ c. leftover **Black Bean and Butternut Squash Chili** (see recipe in Week 1, Wed.), 1 c. pineapple	Mixed vegetables (½ cucumber, 2 oz. baby carrots, ½ c. broccoli) with 2 T. **Goddess Dressing** (see recipe in Week 1, Mon.)	10 oz. **Savory Stuffed Acorn Squash**

SAVORY STUFFED ACORN SQUASH

Serves 4

All the flavors of fall baked into one nutritious dish. Use fresh herbs, if you have them, and breathe in deep to savor the impossibly magical aromas coming from your kitchen.

2 medium acorn squash	¼ c. chopped walnuts
1 t. garlic powder	1 T. soy sauce
½ t. salt	1 t. dried parsley
2 stalks celery, chopped	½ t. dried thyme
1 medium onion, diced	½ t. dried sage
½ c. sliced cremini mushrooms	1 t. salt
2 T. vegan margarine	1 t. black pepper
	½ c. grated vegan cheese

1. Preheat oven to 350°F. Chop squash in half and scrape out any stringy bits and seeds.
2. Sprinkle squash with garlic powder and salt, then place cut-side down on a baking sheet and bake for 30 minutes or until almost soft, then remove from oven.
3. In a large skillet, heat celery, onion, and mushrooms in vegan margarine until soft, about 4–5 minutes.
4. Add walnuts, soy sauce, parsley, thyme, and sage, stirring to combine well, and season with salt and pepper. Heat for another 1–2 minutes until fragrant.
5. Fill squash with mushroom mixture and sprinkle with vegan cheese. Bake another 5–10 minutes until squash is soft.

PER SERVING Calories **284** Fat **17G** Protein **4G** Sodium **1,447MG** Fiber **5G** Carbohydrates **34G** Sugar **7G** Zinc **1MG** Calcium **120MG** Iron **2MG** Vit. D **0MCG** Vit. B$_{12}$ **0MCG**

DID YOU KNOW?

Religious ascetics and philosophers have dabbled with vegetarian and mostly vegan diets throughout history. Among the ancient Greeks, mathematician and philosopher Pythagoras mentored a group of vegetarians in the sixth-century B.C., and until the word *vegetarianism* was coined in the 1840s, diets free from meat and fish were often called "Pythagorean." At the same time in India, the ancient Jains were already practicing ahimsa, pledging not to kill by avoiding animal flesh and eggs.

What I Ate

DATE [   ] | [   ] | [   ]

TIME	FOOD ITEM	AMOUNT	CALORIES	FAT	CARBS	FIBER	PROTEIN
	TOTAL						

Today's Vegan Plate

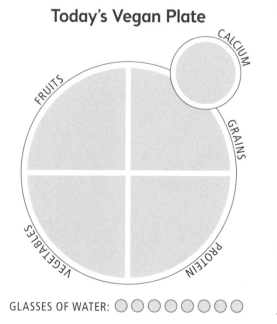

CALCIUM

FRUITS

GRAINS

VEGETABLES

PROTEIN

GLASSES OF WATER: ○○○○○○○○

Thoughts about Today

MENU

BREAKFAST	LUNCH	SNACK	DINNER
1 Strawberry Protein Smoothie (see recipe in Week 2, Tues.), 1 banana	Caesar salad with 2 c. romaine lettuce, 6 oz. vegan chicken, and 1 T. Goddess Dressing (see recipe in Week 1, Mon.); 1 apple; 1 c. orange juice	Mixed fruit salad with ½ apple, ½ banana, ½ c. strawberries, and ½ c. pineapple	5 oz. Garlic Miso and Onion Soup with 1 c. soba noodles, 1 c. steamed spinach with 16g nutritional yeast

GARLIC MISO AND ONION SOUP

Serves 2

This simple soup hits the spot for a light dinner. If you don't have chopped seaweed on hand, simply leave it out.

4 c. water
½ c. sliced shiitake mushrooms
3 scallions, chopped
½ medium yellow onion, chopped
4 cloves garlic, minced
¾ t. garlic powder

2 T. soy sauce
1 t. sesame oil
1 (14-oz.) block silken tofu, diced
⅓ c. miso
1 T. chopped seaweed, any kind

1. Combine all ingredients except miso and seaweed in a large soup or stockpot and bring to a slow simmer. Cook, uncovered, for 10–12 minutes.
2. Reduce heat and stir in miso and seaweed, being careful not to boil.
3. Heat, stirring to dissolve miso, for another 5 minutes until onions and mushrooms are soft.

PER SERVING Calories **245** Fat **10G** Protein **18G** Sodium **1,749MG** Fiber **5G** Carbohydrates **23G** Sugar **6G** Zinc **2G** Calcium **222MG** Iron **4MG** Vit. D **0MCG** Vit. B$_{12}$ **0MCG**

MISO TRIVIA

Miso, a paste made from fermented soybeans, is available in a variety of interchangeable flavors and colors, red, white, and barley miso being the most common. Miso is full of protein and zinc; and because of the fermentation process, miso is rich in enzymes. It's really a personal preference which type you use. Asian grocers stock miso at about a third of the price of natural food stores, so if you're lucky enough to have one in your neighborhood, it's worth a trip. Boiling miso destroys some of its beneficial enzymes, so when making soup, be sure to heat it to just below a simmer.

What I Ate

DATE [   ] | [   ] | [   ]

TIME	FOOD ITEM	AMOUNT	CALORIES	FAT	CARBS	FIBER	PROTEIN
		TOTAL					

Today's Vegan Plate

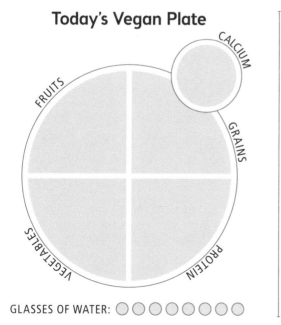

CALCIUM

FRUITS

GRAINS

VEGETABLES

PROTEIN

GLASSES OF WATER: ○○○○○○○○

Thoughts about Today

MENU

BREAKFAST	LUNCH	SNACK	DINNER
6 oz. **Rosemary Tempeh Hash**, 1 c. chocolate soy milk	1½ c. **Black Bean and Butternut Squash Chili** (see recipe in Week 1, Wed.), side green salad with 2 c. romaine lettuce or collard greens, 1 tomato, and 1 diced cucumber, 2 T. **Goddess Dressing** (see recipe in Week 1, Mon.)	200 calories of whole grain chips with ¼ c. **Black Bean Guacamole** (see recipe in Week 2, Tues.)	6 oz. **Easy Three-Bean Casserole**, side green salad with 2 c. romaine lettuce, kale, or spinach, 1 tomato, and 1 diced cucumber, 2 T. **Goddess Dressing** (see recipe in Week 1, Mon.)

ROSEMARY TEMPEH HASH

Serves 4

Rosemary's unique flavor pairs nicely with the scallions and potatoes in this hash. Serve with chopped avocado and hot sauce, if desired.

2 medium red potatoes, diced
Water for boiling
1 (8-oz.) package tempeh, cubed
2 T. olive oil
2 scallions, chopped
1 t. chili powder
1 t. dried rosemary
1 t. salt
1 t. black pepper

1. Cover potatoes with water in a large pot and bring to a boil. Cook just until potatoes are almost soft, about 15 minutes. Drain.
2. In a large pan, sauté potatoes and tempeh in olive oil for 3–4 minutes, lightly browning tempeh on all sides.
3. Add scallions, chili powder, and rosemary, stirring to combine, and heat for 3–4 more minutes. Season with salt and pepper.

PER SERVING Calories **260** Fat **13G** Protein **14G** Sodium **613MG** Fiber **2G** Carbohydrates **25G** Sugar **1G** Zinc **1MG** Calcium **91MG** Iron **3MG** Vit. D **0MCG** Vit. B$_{12}$ **0MCG**

EASY THREE-BEAN CASSEROLE

Serves 8

This bean casserole is packed with protein—and sweet and savory flavors.

1 (15-oz.) can vegan baked beans
1 (15-oz.) can black beans, drained
1 (15-oz.) can kidney beans, drained
1 medium onion, chopped
⅓ c. ketchup
3 T. apple cider vinegar
⅓ c. brown sugar
2 t. mustard powder
2 t. garlic powder
4 vegan hot dogs, cooked and chopped

1. Preheat oven to 350°F.
2. Combine all ingredients except vegan hot dogs in a 9" × 13" casserole dish.
3. Bake for 55 minutes, uncovered. Add precooked vegan hot dogs just before serving.

PER SERVING Calories **215** Fat **1G** Protein **12G** Sodium **666MG** Fiber **7G** Carbohydrates **42G** Sugar **19G** Zinc **2MG** Calcium **78MG** Iron **2MG** Vit. D **0MCG** Vit. B$_{12}$ **0MCG**

What I Ate

DATE | | |

TIME	FOOD ITEM	AMOUNT	CALORIES	FAT	CARBS	FIBER	PROTEIN
TOTAL							

Today's Vegan Plate

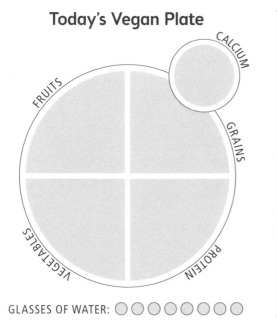

CALCIUM

FRUITS

GRAINS

VEGETABLES

PROTEIN

GLASSES OF WATER: ○○○○○○○○

Thoughts about Today

MENU

BREAKFAST	LUNCH	SNACK	DINNER
2 oz. polenta with ½ c. black beans, 2 slices (1 oz.) vegan cheese	¾ c. Five-Minute Vegan Pasta Salad, 1 banana	1 oz. dried apricots, 1 oz. dried cranberries	5.5 oz. Tofu "Fish" Sticks, 1 steamed sweet potato, 1 ear corn on the cob with 16g nutritional yeast

FIVE-MINUTE VEGAN PASTA SALAD

Serves 4

Once you've got the pasta cooked and cooled, this takes just 5 minutes to assemble, as it's made with store-bought dressing. A balsamic vinaigrette or tomato dressing would also work well.

4 c. cooked pasta
¾ c. vegan Italian salad dressing
3 scallions, chopped
½ c. sliced black olives

1 medium tomato, chopped
1 medium avocado, diced
1 t. salt
1 t. black pepper

Toss together all ingredients. Allow to chill for at least 1½ hours before serving, if time permits, to let flavors combine.

PER SERVING Calories 269 Fat 20G Protein 4G Sodium 1,190MG Fiber 5G Carbohydrates 22G Sugar 6G Zinc 1MG Calcium 33MG Iron 1MG Vit. D 0MCG Vit. B₁₂ 0MCG

INSTANT ADDITIONS

Open up a jar and instantly add color, flavor, and texture to a basic pasta salad. What's in your cupboard? Try capers, roasted red peppers, canned vegetables, jarred pimentos, sun-dried tomatoes, or even mandarin oranges or sliced beets. Slip in any leftover fresh herbs you have on hand.

TOFU "FISH" STICKS

Serves 4

Adding seaweed and lemon juice to baked and breaded tofu gives it a "fishy" taste. Crumbled nori sushi sheets would work well, too, if you can't find kelp or dulse flakes. You could also panfry these "fish" sticks in a bit of oil instead of baking, if you prefer.

½ c. all-purpose flour
⅓ c. unsweetened soy milk
2 T. lemon juice
1½ c. fine ground bread crumbs

2 T. seaweed flakes
1 T. Old Bay seasoning blend
1 t. onion powder
1 (14-oz.) block extra-firm tofu, well pressed

1. Preheat oven to 350°F.
2. Place flour in a shallow bowl or pie tin and set aside. Combine soy milk and lemon juice in a separate shallow bowl or pie tin. In a third bowl or pie tin, combine bread crumbs, seaweed flakes, Old Bay, and onion powder.
3. Slice tofu into ½"-thick strips. Place each strip into the flour mixture to coat well, then dip into the soy milk. Next, place each strip into the bread crumbs, gently patting to coat well.
4. Bake for 15–20 minutes, turn once, then bake for another 10–15 minutes, or until crispy.

PER SERVING Calories 337 Fat 8G Protein 18G Sodium 815MG Fiber 4G Carbohydrates 47G Sugar 3G Zinc 1MG Calcium 182MG Iron 5MG Vit. D 0MCG Vit. B₁₂ 0MCG

What I Ate

DATE [ ] | [ ] | [ ]

TIME	FOOD ITEM	AMOUNT	CALORIES	FAT	CARBS	FIBER	PROTEIN
TOTAL							

Today's Vegan Plate

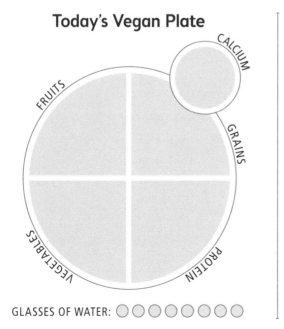

CALCIUM

FRUITS

GRAINS

VEGETABLES

PROTEIN

GLASSES OF WATER: ○○○○○○○○○

Thoughts about Today

REVIEW

I FEEL:

_____
_____
_____
_____
_____

MY GREATEST FOOD DISCOVERY THIS WEEK WAS:

_____
_____
_____
_____
_____

THIS WEEK'S BIGGEST VEGAN CHALLENGE WAS:

_____
_____
_____
_____
_____

NEW FOOD I'D LIKE TO TRY:

_____
_____
_____
_____
_____

WHEN I LOOK BACK AT THIS WEEK, I MOST WANT TO REMEMBER:

_____
_____
_____
_____

HOW ARE YOU PROGRESSING TOWARD YOUR GOALS?

_____
_____
_____
_____

WEEK 12

Being vegan is about so much more than just eating a healthy diet. It's about choosing to live a healthy and compassionate lifestyle; it's about sleeping better at night, knowing your actions are in line with your ethical values; and it's about celebrating all of the life-giving foods that Mother Nature has to offer. This weekend, you will have been vegan for twelve weeks! It's time to celebrate! A few ideas? Cook up your favorite meal, and enjoy it with a lovely bottle of wine (some wines contain animal ingredients, so be sure to choose a vegan wine!). Or venture out and try everything on the menu at the local vegan restaurant. You could also special order a vegan cake, and share it with friends.

But before you do, make sure you're well prepared to continue eating vegan and healthy from here on out on your own. Do you have a plan for Week 13? By now, you should be so comfortable eating vegan that you don't need one. You have plenty of breakfast, lunch, and dinner ideas in your regular repertoire of foods to choose from. If you're still uncertain about getting in all your nutrients, try mixing and matching a few of the meals throughout this planner.

Final words of wisdom? Enjoy a bit of vegan chocolate and vegan ice cream from time to time, and don't forget to get your B_{12}. Welcome to the wonderful world of veganism!

MENU

BREAKFAST	LUNCH	SNACK	DINNER
1 T. peanut butter with 1 T. sugar-free jam on 2 slices whole grain bread, 1 banana	Burrito with 1 large flour tortilla, ½ c. beef substitute, ½ tomato, and ½ c. romaine lettuce; 1 c. tomato juice (no salt added)	Mixed vegetables (½ cucumber, 2 oz. baby carrots, ½ c. broccoli) with 2 T. hummus, 1 oz. cashews	6 oz. Greek Lemon Rice with Spinach and 4½ oz. Lemon Basil Tofu

GREEK LEMON RICE WITH SPINACH

Serves 4

Greek spanakorizo, a soft and creamy Greek dish of spinach and rice, is seasoned with fresh lemon, herbs, and black pepper.

1 medium onion, chopped	2 bunches fresh spinach, trimmed
4 cloves garlic, minced	2 T. chopped fresh parsley
2 T. olive oil	1 T. chopped fresh mint
¾ c. white rice	2 T. lemon juice
2½ c. water	½ t. salt
1 (8-oz.) can tomato paste	½ t. freshly ground black pepper

1. Sauté onions and garlic in olive oil for just 1–2 minutes, then add rice, stirring to lightly toast.
2. Add water, cover, and heat for 10–12 minutes.
3. Add tomato paste, spinach, and parsley. Cover, and cook for another 5 minutes or until spinach is wilted and rice is cooked.
4. Stir in fresh mint, lemon juice, salt, and pepper.

PER SERVING Calories 294 Fat 8G Protein 10G Sodium 420MG Fiber 7G Carbohydrates 50G Sugar 9G Zinc 2MG Calcium 227MG Iron 8MG Vit. D 0MCG Vit. B$_{12}$ 0MCG

A HIGH-PROTEIN RICE?

Wild rice is not actually rice, but rather a seed. With almost 7 grams of protein per cup when cooked, wild rice can be an excellent source of protein, as well as antioxidants. Add ¼ cup wild rice per cup of white rice to any recipe that calls for regular white rice for an extra protein boost.

LEMON BASIL TOFU

Serves 6

Moist and chewy, this zesty baked tofu is reminiscent of lemon chicken. Serve drizzled with extra marinade, or use the extra marinade as a salad dressing.

3 T. lemon juice	3 T. olive oil
1 T. soy sauce	2 T. chopped basil, plus extra for garnish
2 t. apple cider vinegar	2 (14 oz.) blocks extra-firm tofu, well pressed
1 T. Dijon mustard	
¾ t. sugar	

1. Whisk together all ingredients except tofu, and transfer to a baking dish or casserole pan.
2. Slice tofu into ½"-thick strips or triangles.
3. Place tofu in the marinade and coat well. Allow to marinate for at least 1 hour or overnight, being sure tofu is well coated in marinade.
4. Preheat oven to 350°F.
5. Bake for 15 minutes, turn over, then bake for another 10–12 minutes or until done. Garnish with a few extra bits of chopped fresh basil.

PER SERVING Calories 198 Fat 14G Protein 14G Sodium 212MG Fiber 2G Carbohydrates 5G Sugar 1G Zinc 0MG Calcium 106MG Iron 2MG Vit. D 0MCG Vit. B$_{12}$ 0MCG

What I Ate

DATE [   ] | [   ] | [   ]

TIME	FOOD ITEM	AMOUNT	CALORIES	FAT	CARBS	FIBER	PROTEIN
		TOTAL					

Today's Vegan Plate

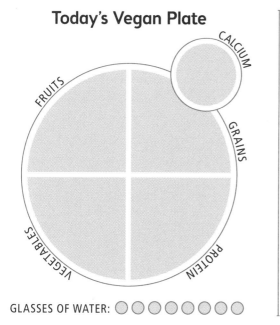

CALCIUM

FRUITS

GRAINS

VEGETABLES

PROTEIN

GLASSES OF WATER: ○○○○○○○○○

Thoughts about Today

BREAKFAST	LUNCH	SNACK	DINNER
1 c. instant grits with 1 (1-oz.) slice vegan cheese, 1 c. unsweetened applesauce	4½ oz. leftover **Greek Lemon Rice with Spinach** and **Lemon Basil Tofu** (see recipes in Week 12, Mon.), 1 apple	1 c. popcorn with 16g nutritional yeast	12 oz. **Fiery Basil and Eggplant Stir-Fry** with 1 c. rice noodles

FIERY BASIL AND EGGPLANT STIR-FRY

Serves 3

Holy basil, called tulsi, is revered in Vishnu temples across India and is frequently used in Ayurvedic healing. Tulsi is commonly used in treatments for high blood pressure, indigestion, high cholesterol, and diabetes, just to name a few. It lends a fantastically spicy flavor, but regular basil will also do.

3 cloves garlic, minced
3 small fresh chili peppers, minced
1 (14-oz.) block extra-firm tofu, pressed and diced
2 T. olive oil
1 medium eggplant, peeled and chopped

1 medium red bell pepper, chopped
⅓ c. sliced shiitake mushrooms
3 T. water
2 T. soy sauce
1 t. lemon juice
⅓ c. fresh tulsi basil

1. Sauté garlic, chili peppers, and tofu in olive oil for 4–6 minutes until tofu is lightly golden.
2. Add eggplant, bell pepper, mushrooms, water, and soy sauce, and heat, stirring frequently, for 5–6 minutes or until eggplant is almost soft.
3. Add lemon juice and basil, and cook for another 1–2 minutes, just until basil is wilted.

PER SERVING Calories **282** Fat **16G** Protein **17G** Sodium **598MG** Fiber **8G** Carbohydrates **19G** Sugar **8G** Zinc **1MG** Calcium **139MG** Iron **3MG** Vit. D **0MCG** Vit. B$_{12}$ **0MCG**

TYPES OF BASIL

Sweet Italian basil may be the most common, but other varieties can add a layer of sensuality enticing flavor. Lemon basil is identifiable by its lighter green color and fresh citrusy scent. For Fiery Basil and Eggplant Stir-Fry, look for spicy holy basil or Thai basil with a purplish stem and jagged leaf edge for a delightfully scorching flavor.

What I Ate

DATE [　　] | [　　] | [　　]

TIME	FOOD ITEM	AMOUNT	CALORIES	FAT	CARBS	FIBER	PROTEIN
	TOTAL						

Today's Vegan Plate

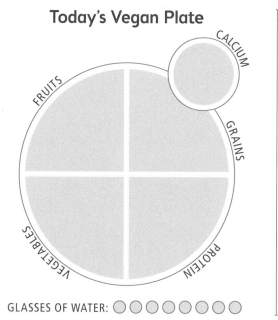

GLASSES OF WATER: ○○○○○○○○○

Thoughts about Today

MENU

BREAKFAST	LUNCH	SNACK	DINNER
1 c. whole grain cereal with ½ c. cashew milk	Grilled cheese sandwich with 2 slices whole grain bread, 2 (1-oz.) slices vegan cheese, 1 c. tomato soup, 1 banana	200 calories of whole grain crackers with 3 T. olive tapenade	1 c. Indian Curried Lentil Soup with 1 c. quinoa

INDIAN CURRIED LENTIL SOUP

Serves 4

Similar to a traditional Indian lentil dal recipe but with added vegetables to make it into an entrée, this lentil soup is perfect as is or perhaps paired with rice or some warmed Indian flatbread.

1 medium onion, diced	1 c. green lentils
1 medium carrot, sliced	2¾ c. vegetable broth
3 whole cloves, minced	2 large tomatoes, chopped
2 T. vegan margarine	1 t. salt
1 t. cumin	¼ t. black pepper
1 t. turmeric	1 t. lemon juice

1. In a large soup or stockpot, sauté onion, carrot, and cloves in margarine until onions are just turning soft, about 3 minutes. Add cumin and turmeric and toast for 1 minute, stirring constantly to avoid burning.
2. Reduce heat to medium low and add lentils, vegetable broth, tomatoes, and salt. Bring to a simmer, cover, and cook for 35–40 minutes, or until lentils are done.
3. Season with black pepper and lemon juice just before serving.

PER SERVING Calories **263** Fat **7G** Protein **14G** Sodium **1,113MG** Fiber **7G** Carbohydrates **39G** Sugar **5G** Zinc **2MG** Calcium **58MG** Iron **4MG** Vit. D **0MCG** Vit. B$_{12}$ **0MCG**

TIME-SAVING SIMMER SAUCES

If you like ethnic food but don't like spending time in the kitchen, an array of vegan simmer sauces is at your fingertips. From Thai curry and satay sauces to Indian masalas, these simmer sauces can be mixed with tofu, vegetables, and a grain for a quick and easy meal. These are usually found in the ethnic foods aisle, but you might also find some near the salad dressings and barbecue sauces.

What I Ate

DATE ☐ | ☐ | ☐

TIME	FOOD ITEM	AMOUNT	CALORIES	FAT	CARBS	FIBER	PROTEIN
TOTAL							

Today's Vegan Plate

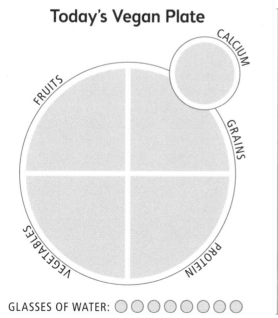

GLASSES OF WATER: ○○○○○○○○

Thoughts about Today

MENU

BREAKFAST	LUNCH	SNACK	DINNER
1 English muffin with 1 vegan sausage patty, ¼ medium tomato (sliced), and 2 oz. avocado slices	1 c. leftover **Indian Curried Lentil Soup** (see recipe in Week 12, Wed.) with 1 slice whole grain toast	1 medium apple with ½ T. peanut butter and ½ oz. raisins, 1 oz. almonds	7 oz. **Creamy Sun-Dried Tomato Pasta**; Greek spinach salad with 2 c. fresh spinach, ½ red bell pepper, 2 T. black olives, ¼ c. chopped artichoke hearts, and 2 T. **Goddess Dressing** (see recipe in Week 1, Mon.)

CREAMY SUN-DRIED TOMATO PASTA

Serves 4

Silken tofu makes a creamy low-fat sauce base. If using dried tomatoes rather than oil-packed, be sure to rehydrate them well first. For another elegant twist on this dish, prepare this recipe with 1¼ cups chopped roasted red peppers instead of sun-dried tomatoes, or try a combination of the two.

1 (12-oz.) package pasta	½ t. garlic powder
1 (14-oz.) block silken tofu, drained	½ t. salt
¼ c. unsweetened soy milk	1¼ c. sun-dried tomatoes, rehydrated
2 T. red wine vinegar	1 t. dried parsley
	2 T. chopped fresh basil

1. Cook pasta according to package instructions and drain well.
2. Blend together tofu, soy milk, vinegar, garlic powder, and salt in a blender or food processor until smooth and creamy. Add tomatoes and parsley and pulse until tomatoes are finely smooth.
3. Transfer sauce to a small pot and heat over medium-low heat just until hot.
4. Pour sauce over pasta and sprinkle with fresh chopped basil.

PER SERVING Calories **424** Fat **5G** Protein **20G** Sodium **589MG** Fiber **6G** Carbohydrates **75G** Sugar **8G** Zinc **1MG** Calcium **129MG** Iron **5MG** Vit. D **0MCG** Vit. B$_{12}$ **0MCG**

ANIMAL AGRICULTURE AFFECTS EVERYONE

The powerful cocktail of hormones and antibiotics pumped into cows and chickens by today's food industry (roughly 70 percent of the antibiotics used in the United States each year are given to animals who are used for food), to make animals grow faster ends up right back in our local water supplies and in the air and affects everyone, even vegans. All these antibiotics, combined with the cramped conditions of modern farms, lead to dangerous new drug-resistant pathogens and bacterial strains. Swine flu, bird flu, SARS, and mad cow disease are all traced back to intense animal agriculture practices. Oh, and don't forget about all of the excrement! A farm with 2,500 dairy cows produces the same amount of waste as a city of 411,000 people, and with animal sewage processing plants, the waste is often stored in "lagoons." According to PETA.org, "Studies have shown that [animal waste] lagoons emit toxic airborne chemicals that can cause inflammatory, immune, irritation, and neurochemical problems in humans."

What I Ate

DATE [   ] | [   ] | [   ]

TIME	FOOD ITEM	AMOUNT	CALORIES	FAT	CARBS	FIBER	PROTEIN
	TOTAL						

Today's Vegan Plate

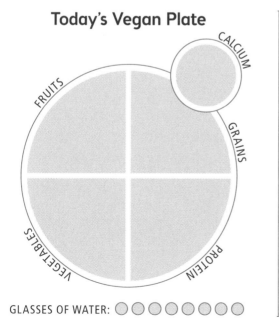

GLASSES OF WATER: ○○○○○○○○

Thoughts about Today

MENU

BREAKFAST	LUNCH	SNACK	DINNER
Breakfast wrap with 1 T. almond butter and ⅓ c. granola in a large flour tortilla, 1 apple, 1 c. orange juice	½ c. baked beans with 1 veggie hot dog, 1 c. pineapple, 1 c. chocolate soy milk	1 pita with 2 T. hummus	10½ oz. No Shepherd, No Sheep Pie

NO SHEPHERD, NO SHEEP PIE

Serves 6

Sheep- and shepherd-less pie is a hearty animal-free entrée for big appetites!

1½ c. TVP
1½ c. hot water
½ medium onion, chopped
2 cloves garlic, minced
1 large carrot, sliced thin
2 t. olive oil
¾ c. sliced button mushrooms
½ c. green peas
½ c. vegetable broth

½ c. plus 3 T. unsweetened soy milk, divided
1 T. all-purpose flour
5 medium Yukon gold potatoes, cooked
2 T. vegan margarine
¼ t. dried rosemary
¼ t. dried sage
½ t. paprika
½ t. salt
¼ t. black pepper

1. Preheat oven to 350°F.
2. Combine TVP and hot water, and allow to sit for 6–7 minutes. Gently drain any excess moisture.
3. In a large skillet, sauté onion, garlic, and carrot in olive oil until onion is soft, about 5 minutes. Add mushrooms, green peas, vegetable broth, and ½ cup soy milk. Whisk in flour just until sauce thickens, then transfer to a casserole dish.
4. Mash together potatoes, margarine, and 3 T. soy milk with rosemary, sage, paprika, salt, and pepper, and spread over the vegetables. Bake for 15 minutes at 350°F.

PER SERVING Calories **303** Fat **6G** Protein **18G** Sodium **326MG** Fiber **8G** Carbohydrates **45G** Sugar **6G** Zinc **1MG** Calcium **152MG** Iron **5MG** Vit. D **0MCG** Vit. B₁₂ **0MCG**

DID YOU KNOW?

According to TheVeganCalculator.com, a vegan personally saves the lives of hundreds of animals a year, reduces her carbon output by an average of 7,300 pounds, conserves 401,500 gallons of water a year, and saves 10,950 square feet of forest. Now that's something to be proud of!

What I Ate

DATE _____ | _____ | _____

TIME	FOOD ITEM	AMOUNT	CALORIES	FAT	CARBS	FIBER	PROTEIN
	TOTAL						

Today's Vegan Plate

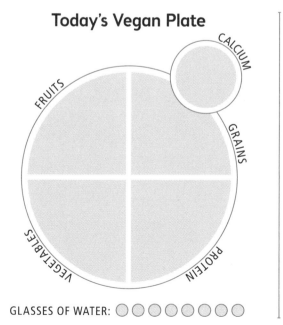

GLASSES OF WATER: ○ ○ ○ ○ ○ ○ ○ ○

Thoughts about Today

MENU

BREAKFAST	LUNCH	SNACK	DINNER
1½ c. **Chili Masala Tofu Scramble** (see recipe in Week 2, Sat.)	Quesadillas with 2 oz. vegan cheese, 2 oz. chicken alternative, and ¼ c. broccoli in a large flour tortilla; ½ c. black beans	Mixed fruit salad with ½ apple, ½ banana, ½ c. strawberries and ½ c. pineapple; 1 granola or energy bar (about 150 calories); 1 oz. cashews	5 oz. **Quick Seitan Teriyaki Chow Mein**

QUICK SEITAN TERIYAKI CHOW MEIN

Serves 2

This veggie-packed dish makes a hearty and nutritious dinner. Garnish with scallions and sesame seeds, if desired.

½ c. seitan, chopped

2 T. olive oil

¼ c. onion, sliced

½ medium green bell pepper, sliced into strips

½ medium red bell pepper, sliced into strips

½ c. broccoli

¾ c. button mushrooms, sliced

½ c. bean sprouts

1 (4-oz.) package chow mein noodles, prepared according to package instructions

2 T. soy sauce

2 T. teriyaki sauce

½ t. dash sesame oil

1. Brown seitan in olive oil for 3–5 minutes, then add onion, peppers, broccoli, and mushrooms and heat, stirring frequently until soft, another 3–5 minutes.
2. Add bean sprouts and allow to cook for 1 minute, then add noodles, soy sauce, teriyaki sauce, and sesame oil, gently mixing to combine. Cook for another minute, just until noodles are heated through.

PER SERVING Calories **555** Fat **24G** Protein **22G** Sodium **2,438MG** Fiber **7G** Carbohydrates **63G** Sugar **14G** Zinc **2MG** Calcium **77MG** Iron **5MG** Vit. D **0MCG** Vit. B$_{12}$ **0MCG**

WHY DO VEGANS LOVE TOFU SO MUCH?

Aside from low cost and ease of preparation, tofu is beloved by many vegans as an excellent source of protein, calcium, and iron. Traditionally an Asian food, plain sautéed tofu with a dash of salt is a quick addition to just about any meal, and many grocery stores offer premarinated and even prebaked tofu that is ready-to-go out of the package. What's more, most tofu brands come in soft, medium, and firm varieties. What's not to love?

What I Ate

DATE [   ] | [   ] | [   ]

TIME	FOOD ITEM	AMOUNT	CALORIES	FAT	CARBS	FIBER	PROTEIN
	TOTAL						

Today's Vegan Plate

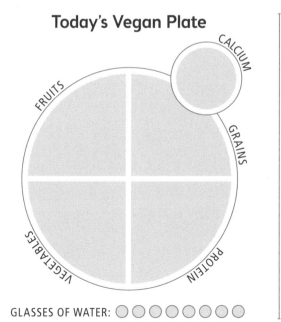

CALCIUM

FRUITS

GRAINS

VEGETABLES

PROTEIN

GLASSES OF WATER: ○○○○○○○○

Thoughts about Today

MENU

BREAKFAST	LUNCH	SNACK	DINNER
Oatmeal breakfast bowl with 1 c. oatmeal, 1 c. blueberries, 1 oz. pecans, and 2 t. maple syrup	**Eggless Egg Salad** sandwich (see recipe in Week 4, Mon.), with ¼ medium tomato, sliced, 2 slices whole grain bread, and ½ c. romaine lettuce, kale, spinach, or sprouts	1 c. **Crispy Baked Kale Chips** (see recipe in Week 5, Sun.)	Your choice! Choose a meal with about 450 calories (or less) and enjoy it with a slice of **Chocolate Peanut Butter Explosion Pie**

CHOCOLATE PEANUT BUTTER EXPLOSION PIE

Serves 8

You can pretend it's healthy because it's made with tofu, or toss away all your troubles to the wind and just enjoy it. You'll feel like a kid again!

¾ c. vegan chocolate chips

1 (12-oz.) block silken tofu

½ c. peanut butter

2 T. unsweetened soy milk

1 prepared vegan cookie piecrust (such as Mrs. Smith's)

1. Over very low heat or in a double boiler, melt chocolate chips.
2. In a blender, purée tofu, peanut butter, and soy milk until combined, then add melted chocolate chips until smooth and creamy.
3. Pour into piecrust and chill for 1 hour, or until firm.

PER SERVING Calories **321** Fat **21G** Protein **8G** Sodium **127MG** Fiber **2G** Carbohydrates **28G** Sugar **12G** Zinc **1MG** Calcium **49MG** Iron **1MG** Vit. D **0MCG** Vit. B$_{12}$ **0MCG**

What I Ate

DATE [ ] | [ ] | [ ]

TIME	FOOD ITEM	AMOUNT	CALORIES	FAT	CARBS	FIBER	PROTEIN
		TOTAL					

Today's Vegan Plate

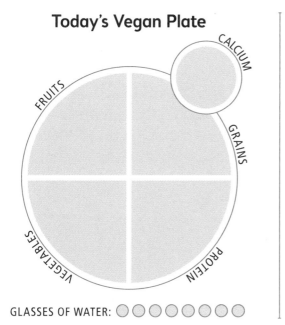

FRUITS

CALCIUM

GRAINS

VEGETABLES

PROTEIN

GLASSES OF WATER: ○○○○○○○○

Thoughts about Today

I FEEL:

MY GREATEST FOOD DISCOVERY THIS WEEK WAS:

THIS WEEK'S BIGGEST VEGAN CHALLENGE WAS:

NEW FOOD I'D LIKE TO TRY:

WHEN I LOOK BACK AT THIS WEEK, I MOST WANT TO REMEMBER:

HOW ARE YOU PROGRESSING TOWARD YOUR GOALS?

INDEX

THE MUST-HAVE VEGAN COOKBOOK FOR THE MUST-HAVE APPLIANCE!

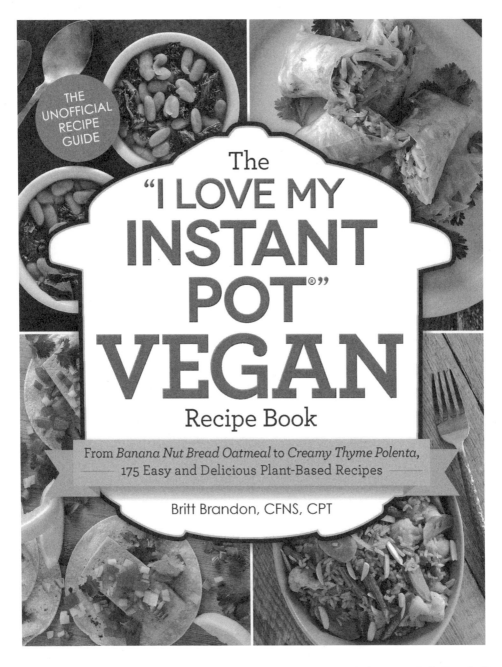

THE UNOFFICIAL RECIPE GUIDE

The "I LOVE MY INSTANT POT®" VEGAN Recipe Book

From *Banana Nut Bread Oatmeal* to *Creamy Thyme Polenta*, 175 Easy and Delicious Plant-Based Recipes

Britt Brandon, CFNS, CPT

PICK UP OR DOWNLOAD YOUR COPY TODAY!

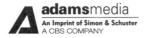

adamsmedia
An Imprint of Simon & Schuster
A CBS COMPANY